Praise for *Yoga by the Stars*

CW00348745

"Jilly's rich and sensitive writing helps us to unpack each of the t
associated color, planet, element, and key qualities … Jilly takes clas:
sequences them creatively and thoughtfully to reflect the essence of ᵕ
tice is clearly explained and illustrated, with different options offered throughout to make the
postures as strong or as gentle as you need them to be … The writing is intelligent and thought-
provoking, every page holding a new insight or reflection … This book is an absolute gem."

—Judy Brenan, British Wheel of Yoga teacher
and foundation course tutor

"Jilly Shipway has brought the power of zodiac imagery to yoga in a way that is engaging, accessible and powerful … There's a wealth of knowledge in this book, presented in a fun yet thought-
provoking style. The practices are clear yet deep, brimming with ideas … This is a fabulous book,
one to treasure and plunder regularly."

—Deana Morris, editor of *Spectrum* magazine and yoga teacher

"In combining astrology with yoga, Jilly Shipway has created a thought-provoking and fun new
way to enjoy these ancient arts. *Yoga by the Stars* assigns each of the twelve zodiac signs a mix-
ture of themes, yoga sequences, affirmations, chants, visualizations, and meditations. Whatever
your sign, each chapter has a relevance and is peppered with little nuggets of philosophy, spar-
kling gems of wisdom, and jewel-like challenges, which have surprised and delighted."

—Linda Poole, yoga student and astrology enthusiast

"This delightful book describes a wonderful link between the two ancient practices of yoga and
astrology, using this connection as an aid to our daily yoga practice and meditation … I love the
idea of using the properties of each sign to inspire yoga practices, to encourage visualizations,
and to cultivate affirmations."

—Jill Carr, experienced yoga student and astrologer

"*Yoga by the Stars* is an ingenious way of creatively combining ancient and modern teachings
(with documentation) on yoga, astrology, meditation, astronomy, guided imagery, and more.
The practices given by Jilly Shipway are clear, accessible, and thoughtful. They are as practical as
they are inspiring. Simultaneously, they will plant your feet on the ground, compassionately lift
and open your heart, and embrace your soul with grace and wonderment. Overall, your understanding of yourself, others, and of the universe we share will expand beautifully."

—Julie Lusk, author of *Yoga Nidra Meditations*

"*Yoga by the Stars* is a fascinating, highly original read for anyone interested in yoga and/or astrology. It doesn't matter if you know a lot or a little about either subject. It's a joy to read and follow, but its beguiling simplicity belies a greater depth and breadth. It's a book you can read straight through, dip into, or pick and mix. It works on so many levels in so many ways. There's something for everyone."

—Lindy Roy, viniyoga teacher

"Through years of her own personal exploration, Jilly Shipway has crafted a series of simple and accessible yoga practices that invite us into our own exploration of the symbols and archetypes that inspired our ancestors … This book will be a gift for your intuitive heart."

—Summer Cushman, MDiv, E-RYT500, C-IAYT,
creator of the Yoga Church Sunday Sermons

"Jilly has created an essential and transformative toolkit for teachers and practitioners of yoga alike. This wonderful book contains straightforward but powerful practices that evoke the essence of each zodiac sign … Jilly skillfully weaves yogic philosophy and practices together with thought-provoking visualizations and meditation questions to explore the turn of the zodiac wheel within oneself … This book is a treasure and a gift for those wishing for greater harmony with themselves."

—Jill Amison, senior yoga teacher and empowerment leader

"Jilly once again brings a deeper meaning to the knowledge that everything is connected. This book offers up to the yoga community various ways to weave astrological elements into our variety of yoga practices. I particularly enjoyed the challenge in the use of associating gender to the sun and moon yoga practices and alternatives. Jilly embodies wonderfully the phrase, 'Earth below, sky above, and peace within.'"

—Lindsey Porter, yoga tutor and author of
Whirlpools, Yoga and the Balance of Life

"Jilly Shipway invites us to deepen our personal journeys with zodiac-inspired yoga practices. By bringing together the wisdom of the zodiac with the self-discovery practices of the yoga tradition, *Yoga by the Stars* is a unique approach to deepen self-awareness and support transformation. This book is rich in knowledge about astrology and offers a variety of yoga movement and meditation practices as well as affirmations to lead you to your inner starlight."

—Jennifer Kreatsoulas, PhD, C-IAYT, founder of
Yoga for Eating Disorders and author of *Body Mindful Yoga*

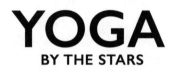

YOGA

BY THE STARS

About the Author

Jilly Shipway is a writer and a qualified yoga teacher. She is the author of *Yoga Through the Year: A Seasonal Approach to Your Practice.*

Jilly has more than twenty-five years of teaching experience. Over her long teaching career, she has enthused hundreds of students with her love of yoga, and many of them have continued to study with her for many years and up to the present day. She has tutored foundation level, pre-diploma yoga study courses for the British Wheel of Yoga. She was very fortunate to have discovered yoga in her early teens and so has had a lifetime of studying and practicing yoga. Mindfulness is an integral part of her own yoga practice and her teaching.

As well as teaching general yoga classes, she also has many years of experience teaching specialist yoga classes to adults recovering from mental health problems. She trained at King's College London as a motivational interviewing coach, coaching people caring for someone with an eating disorder, and worked under the supervision of Professor Janet Treasure and her team.

Jilly's original motivation to write was a curiosity about the mystery of women's involvement (and apparent absence) in the historical evolution of yoga. It was her research into this subject that led her, in a roundabout way, to develop a seasonal approach to yoga and to study astrology. For the past ten years, Jilly has been studying the zodiac wheel and creating zodiac-inspired yoga practices, as well as teaching popular Zodiac Yoga courses. She has a BA (Hons) in fine art and believes passionately that yoga and mindfulness can really enhance creativity.

Jilly regularly contributes to various magazines and yoga publications. When she is not teaching, writing about, or doing yoga, she loves walking in town and country and, of course, gazing at the night sky. She lives in the UK in a small Welsh border town, surrounded by hills. She is married and has one grown-up daughter.

Visit her websites at www.yogabythestars.com or www.yogathroughtheyear.com.

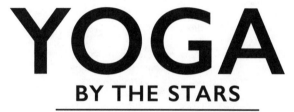

YOGA

BY THE STARS

Practices and Meditations Inspired by the Zodiac

JILLY SHIPWAY

Llewellyn Publications
Woodbury, Minnesota

FIRST EDITION
First Printing, 2020

Cover design by Shannon McKuhen
Interior yoga illustrations by Llewellyn Art Department, based on art by Jilly Shipway
Chakra illustration on page 29 © Mary Ann Zapalac

Llewellyn is a registered trademark of Llewellyn Worldwide Ltd.

Library of Congress Cataloging-in-Publication Data
Names: Shipway, Jilly, author.
Title: Yoga by the stars : practices and meditations inspired by the zodiac
  / Jilly Shipway.
Description: First edition. | Woodbury, Minnesota : Llewellyn Publications,
  [2020] | Includes bibliographical references. | Summary: "A yearlong
  series of yoga practices inspired by the zodiac and each sign's
  symbolism"— Provided by publisher.
Identifiers: LCCN 2020034202 (print) | LCCN 2020034203 (ebook) | ISBN
  9780738763866 (paperback) | ISBN 9780738764252 (ebook)
Subjects: LCSH: Yoga. | Zodiac—Health aspects. | Self-consciousness
  (Awareness) | Self-actualization (Psychology)
Classification: LCC RA781.67 .S47 2020 (print) | LCC RA781.67 (ebook) |
  DDC 613.7/046—dc23
LC record available at https://lccn.loc.gov/2020034202
LC ebook record available at https://lccn.loc.gov/2020034203

Llewellyn Publications
A Division of Llewellyn Worldwide Ltd.
2143 Wooddale Drive
Woodbury, MN 55125-2989
www.llewellyn.com

Printed in the United States of America

Also by Jilly Shipway

Yoga Through the Year: A Seasonal Approach to Your Practice

For Margaret Hone, my stellar guide
For Simon, my willow

Disclaimer

Before beginning any new exercise program, it is recommended that you seek medical advice from your healthcare provider. You have full responsibility for your safety and should know your limits. Before practicing asana poses as described in this book, be sure that you are well informed of proper practice and do not take risks beyond your experience and comfort levels. The publisher and the author assume no liability for any injuries caused to the reader that may result from the reader's use of the content contained herein and recommend common sense when contemplating the practices described in the work.

Contents

Exercises

Yoga Practices

Meditations and Visualizations

Acknowledgments

A huge thank-you to the team at Llewellyn, who have worked on this book and made it the best that it can be. Thank you to my editor, Angela Wix, for steering the book in the best possible direction. I have benefited so much from her unerringly good judgment and experience. Thanks go to my production editor, Lauryn Heineman, for her warmth, patience, and always pertinent corrections to my work. Thanks also to Lynne Menturweck for sensitively interpreting and reproducing my hand-drawn yoga pin people; to the book's designer, Donna Burch-Brown; to Kat Sanborn and Anna Levine for their wonderful work on behalf of the book; and to Shannon McKuhen for bringing the book to life with such a beautiful cover.

Thanks to my daughter, Kay, for all the inspiring conversations we've had about yoga and astrology over the years, as well as for all the fun, laughter, and happiness you bring to my life.

Thanks to my husband, Simon, for lightening my load and freeing me up to write this book. Thanks for hugs, hot drinks, delicious meals, stargazing, and all the laughter and love we share together.

Thanks so much to my family and friends—sorry not to mention you all by name, but your love and friendship mean a lot to me. During the long process of writing this book, it has been such a tonic to go out for country walks with you, share meals, swap texts, share jokes, and have fun together.

Thanks to all the yoga students who have attended my Zodiac Yoga courses; your feedback and enthusiasm have really helped me shape the ideas presented in this book. Thanks also to my many loyal, local students who have studied with me over many years. Your enthusiasm for yoga inspires me and makes teaching a joy.

I'm grateful for the friendship and support of the yoga community, both locally and, thanks to the internet, all over the world. Thanks to Judy Brenan for always going the extra mile. I continue to draw inspiration from teachers such as Sandra Sabatini, Donna Farhi, Sarah Powers, Judith Lasater, and the late Vanda Scaravelli.

Thanks to Zanna Frearson for a wonderfully timely reading list for Jung's studies in astrology and for so generously arranging for the books to be sent to me!

Thank you to Margaret E. Hone, the astrologer, for shining a light onto the twelve signs of the zodiac and revealing them to me in all their rainbow colors.

*It is impossible to affirm with assurance why these twelfths of the Zodiac
seem to be like twelve different colored windows
through which a shining white light is unmistakably varied.*
—Margaret E. Hone, *The Modern Text-Book of Astrology*

———

*Whatever is born or done this moment of time
has the quality of this moment of time.*
—Carl G. Jung

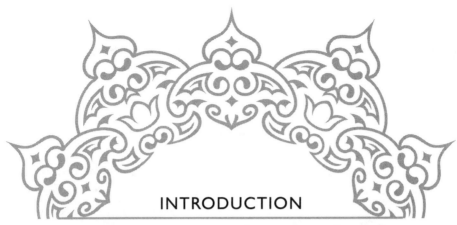

Yoga Inspired by the Stars

The earth and her changing seasons provided the inspiration for my first book, *Yoga Through the Year: A Seasonal Approach to Your Practice*. At the same time as I was researching and writing that book, I was also creating yoga practices that were inspired by looking up at the stars.

Since ancient times women and men have felt a sense of wonder when they looked up at the night sky. Joining the dots of a group of stars fired up their imagination, and they envisioned them as animal shapes and mystical objects. They told stories about these constellations, and these became myths that were handed down through time. Across the globe, over millennia, the learning that has been garnered by stargazing has been formulated into zodiacal systems. When we tap into these systems, we gain access to an ancient wisdom and mythology. It is this celestial wisdom, its stories, and its symbols that I have drawn upon as inspiration for the yoga practices and meditations in this book.

Yoga by the Stars Is for Everyone

I discovered yoga in my early teens, and so I've had a lifetime of studying and practicing yoga. I've been teaching yoga for more than twenty-five years, and for more than ten years I have been studying astrology and integrating the richness of the symbolism contained within the zodiac wheel into my own yoga practice and teaching. I have found that delving into the zodiac treasure chest has taken me on a magical journey that has deepened and enriched my life and my understanding of yoga. The many students I have worked with over the years report back that their experience of working in this way has been transformative too.

Whereas some astrologers use astrology to predict character and destiny, my own interest lies more in viewing the twelve zodiac signs as twelve archetypal personalities who are universally recognized and resonate with something deep in our psyche. By connecting with these twelve archetypal characters, we are connecting to an ancient lore and wisdom. Consequently, my approach to astrology means that the star-inspired yoga practices and meditations in this book can be enjoyed by everyone regardless of their views on astrology.

Over my years of study, practice, and teaching of yoga and astrology, I have developed a method of creating yoga practices that are inspired by a specific zodiac sign but are not designed exclusively to be used by those who happen to be born under that sign. In turn this means that the twelve Zodiac Yoga practices in this book are suitable for everyone, regardless of what sign they are. My intention is to make the healing power of these zodiac-inspired yoga practices available to all regardless of their birth sign or belief system.

Study the zodiac signs and you will see aspects of your own personality reflected in all the signs. When you combine this astrological study with yoga, the result is an increased self-awareness and self-knowledge. Yoga and your zodiac exploration will enable you to shine the light of awareness into the depths of your unconscious and bring into the light your strengths, weaknesses, hidden complexes, and compulsions, as well as reveal any hidden forces that are exerting a gravitational pull upon you and skewing your natural path of orbit. Once out in the light, you have a chance to find ways of resolving these difficulties. You can untie and untangle the knots of your complexes and remove the boulders that are strewn along your way. In turn this will lead you onto the path of healing, transformation, and freedom.

The Healing Power of the Zodiac

The zodiac-inspired yoga practices that I have created for this book have the potential to bring healing and transformation into your life regardless of your own Sun sign. Consequently, you can use all the practices as spiritual medicine to help you to balance and retune your lunar and solar energies.

Below is a guide to the healing potential offered by each of the zodiac signs. The signs will be described in more detail later in the zodiac chapters of this book:

Aries: Empower your inner warrior, reignite your fiery energy, and reconnect with your assertive, courageous and confident self.

Taurus: Fulfill your potential, live with passion, bring beauty and sensual enjoyment into your life, and uncover hidden talents—blossom!

Gemini: Transcend limitations, ignite your spark of genius, reconcile opposing parts of yourself, unite your heaven and earth energies, and let your spirit fly higher!

Cancer: Create your sanctuary, find respite from the fray of life, nurture and nourish yourself, attend to your inner child, and take time out for healing. Relax into the support that life can offer.

Leo: Develop fierce confidence and voice your truth with your lion's roar! Own your expertise, connect with your powerful Sun-self, and radiate your light out into the world. Build powerful, cooperative connections with others.

Virgo: Discover your radiant, authentic self. Know yourself and bat away false assumptions made by others. Find purity by honoring who you truly are. Find healing through working for a pure planet for all to enjoy.

Libra: Open to the wisdom of your heart, restore peace to a troubled mind, and learn to live harmoniously and in a state of equilibrium. Reconcile pairs of opposites in your life so that healing may occur. Make judgments, take action, and create a more peaceful, harmonious world for all.

Scorpio: Face fear and find freedom and transformation. Learn to listen for the still, small voice of calm that will guide you through the storms of life. Shine the light of kind and loving attention to illuminate the dark spaces of the mind.

Sagittarius: Develop the power of clear intention to create miracles in your life. Learn to connect to a spacious, open, and expansive awareness by narrowing and focusing your attention. Take new paths, travel far, laugh, love, and live life to the fullest.

Capricorn: Transcend limitations and find liberation. Find new ways of working with and overcoming restrictions in your life. Discover the opportunities that lie dormant within your difficulties and open the door to self-discovery.

Aquarius: Draw from the wellspring of love. Learn the art of kind, compassionate detachment. Be rebellious, be generous, dance, and ride the waves of change. Combine science, creativity, and love to bring healing to the world.

Pisces: Dive deep to find self-knowledge. Peep behind the veil of the subconscious mind and free yourself from hidden influences and unwelcome gravitational pulls. Become the Sun at the center of your own life. Attune yourself to the circular flow of life and learn to welcome light and dark, waxing and waning, and come face to face with love.

The Treasures of the Zodiac Revealed

The zodiac signs provide a direct link to our ancestors, their world, and how they perceived the cosmos. Over millennia almost all cultures have projected their lives and concerns onto the stars. As they gazed up at the night sky, dramas were played out, reflecting the story of their own lives here on earth. Also, if you bear in mind the fact that we are literally made from the stuff of stars, then it follows that whatever we project onto the stars has its origin in the stars and consequently will potentially encapsulate universal, cosmological truths. Just as Western astrologers may quote the Hermetic axiom, "As above, so below," the Tantric yogis put it the other way around: "As in the body, so in the universe."[1]

In this book, *Yoga by the Stars*, we take a pilgrimage around the wheel of the zodiac. It's a journey through space and time and an exploration of how the constellation of your personality, your world, and the cosmos interact with time, the seasons, and a constantly changing universe. The Irish poet Louis MacNeice, in his book *Astrology*, puts forward the theory that a pilgrimage around the zodiac is an evolution from the material to the spiritual, ending in the state of yoga: "The first six signs, beginning with Aries … represent the achievement of full objective consciousness … and the latter (or homeward?) six represent 'evolution into the subjective states, or yoga.' The twelfth sign Pisces corresponds to the ascension into heaven."[2]

To make the most of your journey around the zodiac, keep in mind the image of yourself as the sun at the center and the signs as the planets orbiting around you. The

---

1. Valerie J. Roebuck, *The Circle of Stars: An Introduction to Indian Astrology* (Rockport, MA: Element, 1992), 12.

2. Louis MacNeice, *Astrology* (London: Bloomsbury, 1989), 77.

zodiac signs are your teachers, but it is your light that illuminates the lessons and provides the energy for change to occur.

The twelve zodiac chapters in this book are the fruit of my many years of pilgrimaging around the zodiac and finding inspiration therein to create zodiac-inspired yoga practices and meditations. They have been tried and tested over time by me and the many students who have attended my Zodiac Yoga courses. I believe that within each of the zodiac signs is a gift waiting to be unwrapped. There is a gift for everyone regardless of their beliefs about astrology. My quest has been to uncover the treasures of yoga, which are the gift to be found within each sign, and to share them with you in each of the chapters of this book. Yoga's treasures are like an eternal spring, perpetual and forever being replenished and renewed. I am privileged to have been bestowed these gems to share with you.

How to Use This Book

This section will give you some tips on how to get the most out of this book and how to navigate your way around it. After you've read this section, move on to chapter 1, "The Yoga by the Stars Practice," where you'll learn more about the elements that are found in each of the zodiac chapters and how best to work with them. I'd suggest you also read chapter 2, "Yoga and the Wheel of the Zodiac," to familiarize yourself with the astrological approach and tools that are used in the book. After that you're ready to dive into the astrological and zodiac sign chapters.

Each chapter contains the following elements:

- The zodiac chapters begin with an introduction that reflects on the yoga wisdom that is encapsulated within the zodiac sign for that month. These are written in such a way that the zodiac sign is not specifically mentioned so that the treasure found within the sign is universal and relevant to everyone regardless of their beliefs about astrology. If you already know a lot about astrology, you might enjoy doing some detective work to see if you can spot the zodiac themes that are embedded but hidden in all the chapter's introductions. This is followed with a look at the astrological themes that have inspired the yoga practice for the month's sign.
- Next up is a yoga practice inspired by the month's sign. Integrated into each yoga practice is an affirmation that has the wisdom of the sign's theme condensed into a short, inspiring phrase.

- The yoga practice is followed by a meditation, visualization, breathing practice, or relaxation, all of which are related to and inspired by the sign's yoga theme for the month.
- Each of the zodiac sign chapters concludes with a set of meditation questions related to the theme for the month. Working with these questions will help you explore the theme, gain insights relevant to your own life, and so bring about transformation and healing.

The book is circular in nature, so each chapter functions as an independent entity and at the same time is an essential part of the constellation of chapters that form this book. Remember that, regardless of what Sun sign you are, the zodiac sign chapters of the book are universally relevant to everyone. If you like a particular zodiac chapter, it's fine to return to its wisdom and practices at any time of the year. I hope you make the book and its practices your own and use them in a way that helps you shine.

PART 1

The Yoga by the Stars Approach

CHAPTER 1

The Yoga by the Stars Practice

When you come to reading the zodiac-inspired chapters, you'll find most of the elements in the chapter need no explanation. However, to help you make the most of the book, I'd like to give you a few simple guidelines for working with the yoga practices, the affirmations, and the meditation questions contained within each chapter.

The Yoga Asana Practices

The zodiac-inspired yoga practices that I have created for this book are simple, accessible, and easy to use. You don't need to be hyperflexible or super fit to use them, although using them will improve your flexibility and general fitness.

The yoga practices are easy to follow and use, with each pose accompanied by a simple illustration and clear instructions. The English and Sanskrit names are given for each of the yoga poses (*asanas*) used in the book, so if you want more information about a yoga pose, just do a quick internet search using the pose name. If you are new to yoga and unfamiliar with the poses described, think about attending a class to allow you to learn the positions correctly.

If you are an experienced yoga practitioner, I feel confident that if you choose to, you'll be able to adapt my yoga practices to increase their intensity, substituting stronger poses if required. Mindfulness practitioners could use the yoga practices in this book as the mindful movement component of their regular mindfulness practice.

I'd like to encourage you to make the yoga practices in this book your own. Trying out a new yoga practice is like trying out a new recipe. The first few times you attempt a new recipe, if you're like me, you'll follow the instructions to a tee, weighing out exact amounts, sticking to the recommended ingredients and cooking times, and so on. Once you feel more confident about the dish, you'll add more or less sugar or salt, seasoning, spices; add a new ingredient; and so on. It's the same with your yoga: once you've tried a new yoga practice a few times, you can use your imagination, creativity, ingenuity, and intuition to spice up or tone down the practice. Trust your instinct and make the practices your own—that's what *Yoga by the Stars* is all about!

Beginning and Ending Your Yoga Session: Warming Up and Winding Down

Below you will find a yoga warm-up that you can use to prepare for the yoga practices in this book. There is also a yoga Wind-Down Routine that you can use to follow the yoga practices in this book.

Universal Warm-Up Routine

The routine below can be used to prepare for the yoga practices in this book. It takes about 8 to 10 minutes. If you're pushed for time, it can also be used on its own as a mini yoga practice. It's a great wake-me-up first thing in the morning, preparing you for the day ahead and boosting your mood. At the end of these instructions you'll find an illustrated aide-mémoire for the whole practice.

1. Walking on the spot with arm raises

Stand tall, feet hip width apart. Walk on the spot. As you walk, on the inhale raise the arms out to the side and above the the head; on the exhale lower them back to sides. Repeat 6 times.

Walking on the spot with arm raises

2. Bend and straighten warm-up

Take the legs 2 to 3 feet apart and turn the toes slightly out. Take the arms out to the sides at shoulder height, palms facing downward. On your next exhale, bend the knees and lower the arms. Inhale, return to the starting position. Repeat 6 times.

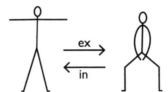

Bend and straighten warm-up

3. Dynamic Side Bend

Legs are 2 to 3 feet apart, toes turned slightly out, arms by your side. Inhale as you bend your right knee and raise your left arm overhead into a side-bend to the right. Exhale, lower the arm, and straighten the leg, returning to the starting position. Repeat 6 times. On the final time stay for a few breaths in the side bend. Repeat on the other side.

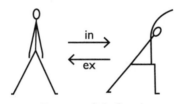

Dynamic Side Bend

4. Dynamic Horse Pose (Vatayanasana) variation

With legs apart, toes turned slightly out, take both arms out to the side and above your head, bringing the hands together. Exhaling, bend both knees, as if you were sitting down on a high stool, bringing the hands to the heart in prayer position. Inhaling, straighten the legs, taking arms out to the side and above the head, back to the starting position. Repeat 4 times. On the final time stay for a few breaths in the Dynamic Horse Pose (*Vatayanasana*) variation.

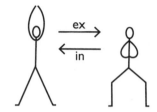

Dynamic Horse Pose variation

5. *Walking on the spot with arm raises*

Stand tall, feet hip width apart. Walk on the spot. As you walk, on the inhale raise the arms out to the side and above the the head; on the exhale lower them back to sides. Repeat 6 times.

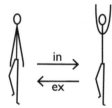

Walking on the spot with arm raises

Universal Warm-Up Routine Overview

1. Walking on the spot with arm raises × 6.

2. Bend and straighten warm-up × 6.

3. Dynamic Side-Bend × 6. On final time stay for a few breaths. Repeat on other side.

4. Dynamic Horse Pose variation × 4. On final time stay for a few breaths.

5. Walking on the spot with Arm Raises × 6.

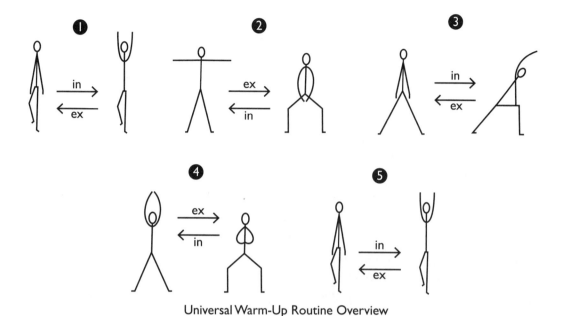

Universal Warm-Up Routine Overview

Universal Wind-Down Routine

This Universal Wind-Down Routine can be used to follow the yoga practices in this book, and it will help you to return to a neutral, relaxed, pre-exercise state. It could also be used on its own as a mini yoga practice when you are pushed for time. It's particularly good as a relaxing practice at the end of the day. It takes about 10 to 12 minutes. At the end of these instructions you'll find an illustrated aide-mémoire for the whole practice.

1. Supine Twist (Jathara Parivrtti) *modified*

Lie on your back, knees bent, feet together, arms out to the sides at shoulder height, and palms facing down. Bring both knees onto your chest (for an easier pose keep both feet on the floor). Exhaling, lower both knees down toward the floor on the left; turn your head gently to the right. Inhale and return to center. Repeat 6 times on each side, alternating sides, and then stay in the pose for a few breaths on each side.

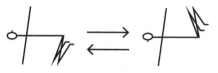

Supine Twist modified

2. Curl-Up with leg raises

Bring the knees into the chest, hands holding the back of the thighs. Exhale and curl the head and shoulders off the floor to look along the midline of the body; from here straighten legs up toward the ceiling. While inhaling, bend the knees back into the chest and lower head and shoulders back to the floor. Repeat 4 times.

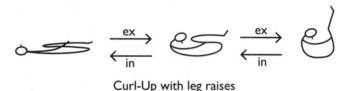

Curl-Up with leg raises

3. Bridge Pose with arm movements (Setu Bandhasana)

Lie on your back with both knees bent, feet on the floor hip width apart, and arms by your sides. Inhale and peel the back from the floor, coming up into Bridge Pose (*Setu Bandhasana*), while simultaneously taking the arms up above the head and onto the floor behind you. Exhale and return to the starting position. Repeat 6 times.

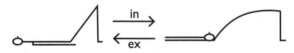

Bridge Pose with arm movements

4. Knee Circles

Bring the knees onto the chest, one hand resting lightly on each kneecap. Keeping the hands on the knees, take the knees out to the side away from you and then back together (drawing a figure eight with the knees). Repeat 6 times, and then 6 times in the opposite direction.

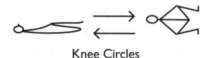

Knee Circles

5. Supine Butterfly Pose (Supta Baddha Konasana) variation

Lie on your back with the knees on your chest, one hand cupping the outside of each knee. Allow the knees to fall out to the sides as wide as is comfortable. For more of a stretch, take the hands to take hold of the inner lower leg and let the big toes move away from each other. Stay here for a few breaths, relaxing into the pose. With each inhale imagine that you are taking the breath all the way down to the pelvic floor; with each exhale gently pull in and up the muscles of the pelvic floor.

Supine Butterfly Pose

6. Leg Stretch Sequence

Bring both knees onto your chest. Inhale and straighten your legs vertically, heels toward the ceiling, and take your arms out to the side just below shoulder height, palms facing up. Exhale and bring your knees back to your chest and hands back to your knees. Next time around, inhale, straighten your legs vertically, and take your arms over your head and onto the floor behind you. Repeat the sequence 6 times, alternating arm movements.

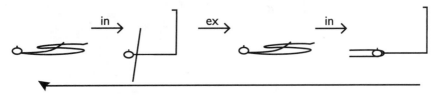

Leg Stretch Sequence

7. Full-Body Stretch

Lying on your back, stretch both legs out along the floor and take both arms overhead. Lengthen tall along the floor. Stay for a few breaths.

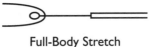

Full-Body Stretch

8. Rest

Rest for a few breaths with knees bent and feet on the floor, hip width apart.

You can either finish your practice here, or if you are using this Universal Wind-Down Routine as part of one of the zodiac-inspired yoga practices, you can continue with that practice and do their suggested meditation or relaxation.

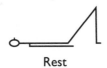

Rest

Universal Wind-Down Routine Overview

1. Supine Twist × 6 on each side, alternating sides.
2. Curl-Up with leg raises × 4.
3. Bridge Pose with arm movements × 6.
4. Knee Circles × 6 each way.
5. Supine Butterfly Pose variation. Stay a few breaths.
6. Leg Stretch Sequence × 6 rounds.
7. Full-Body Stretch.
8. Rest for a few breaths.

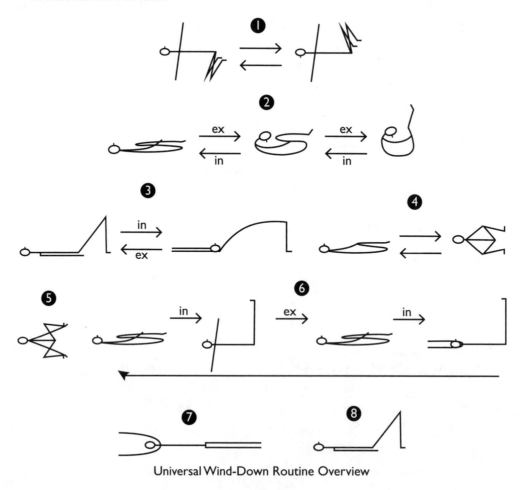

Universal Wind-Down Routine Overview

How to Use the Affirmations in Each Chapter

The affirmations relate to the chapter's zodiac-inspired yoga theme and condense it down into one short inspirational phrase. They are a simple and effective way of steering yourself in the direction of developing positive qualities and attitudes. For example, for the Aries chapter the affirmation is *I am filled with love and courage*. Repetition of this phrase gently opens your mind to the idea that love and courage are possibilities for you.

The affirmations are integrated into the monthly yoga practices included in each chapter of this book, and they can be used in a variety of ways:

Silently repeat them at any time during the day to uplift and inspire. Say them just before going to bed in the evening or upon waking in the morning. For example, when you wake up in the morning, you could repeat the affirmation *I am filled with love and courage* three times, and this would set a loving and courageous tone for the day. You could also repeat it just before you go to bed, and then it will be working in your subconscious overnight.

They can be repeated a few times at the start and end of your yoga practice or silently repeated while you hold a yoga pose. When you step onto your yoga mat, you could begin your practice with the affirmation. Then, when you are holding a pose, you could repeat, *I am filled with love and courage*. The shortened version of the affirmations can be coordinated with the breath as a meditation or used when you are coordinating dynamic yoga movements with the breath. If you're using a pose dynamically by, for example, raising the arms on the inhalation and lowering on the exhalation, you could say *love* as you raise the arms and *courage* as you lower them.

At the end of the session, just before you go into relaxation, repeat the affirmation a few more times. During your relaxation, you could silently repeat the words *love* and *courage* coordinated with a slow, relaxed breathing pattern as a meditative way of focusing and calming the mind.

Each of the chapter's affirmations can be used during that sign's month or at any other time if it feels right to you.

How to Use the Meditation Questions

The meditation questions help you explore the zodiac-inspired yoga themes for the month. They are simple to use and can easily be fitted into your day. They are a way of accessing your own inner life coach and helping you gain access to the wisdom of your subconscious. They build your confidence in your ability to create change and transformation in your life.

To give you an idea of how to use the meditation questions, let's have a look at one. For example, in the Aries chapter, we are developing the theme of building courage. One of the meditation questions in this chapter is "What qualities would I possess if I were a spiritual warrior?" You could work with this question in the following ways:

- In the evening at bedtime pose the question, and then overnight let your subconscious mind get to work on coming up with some answers to it.
- Pose the question while out walking or during a walking meditation. Gently turn the question over in your mind; you don't need to chase the answers.
- Use the question as your focus during a sitting meditation. If your mind wanders off, gently bring it back to the question and your mind's response to it.
- Use the question as your focus for a writing meditation. Set your timer for 5 to 20 minutes and just write down whatever comes into your head in response to the question. No need to worry about spelling, grammar, handwriting, and so on. Just keep the pen on the paper and keep writing.
- Pose the question at the beginning or end of your yoga session during a period of Relaxation Pose (*Savasana*), or repeat it silently while you are holding a yoga pose and relaxing into it.

Whichever way you choose to use the meditation questions, be prepared for magic to happen in your life!

Now, I'd suggest that you read the following two chapters, "Yoga and the Wheel of the Zodiac" and "The Sun, the Moon, Yoga, and You," in order to find out more about the astrological approach and tools used in this book and to astrologically orient yourself. After that, you are ready to dive into the zodiac-inspired chapters in the rest of the book. I wish you an uplifting and inspiring interstellar journey through the zodiac signs and yoga.

CHAPTER 2

Yoga and the Wheel of the Zodiac

This chapter will help you to familiarize yourself with the astrological approach and tools that are used in this book. I'll also introduce you to some of the zodiac concepts that are woven into each of the chapters of the book. We'll look at some unconventional and creative ways of working with the zodiac signs and how to use them as a springboard to inspire your yoga practice and enrich your life.

How I Create Yoga Practices Inspired by the Zodiac

At first sight yoga and astrology might seem an unconventional pairing. However, my method of creating yoga practices inspired by the zodiac has always remained true to the yoga tradition I was trained in and that I have spent the best part of my lifetime studying. Yoga and meditation teach you to train your awareness to focus on the "object" of meditation. Over several years, the zodiac wheel has been my object of meditation, and I have shone the light of my awareness onto it and interrogated it. This may sound a bit intense—well, at times it has been, but also at other times it's been really good fun and always rewarding.

The techniques that I have used to explore the zodiac wheel and to relate it back to yoga are walking meditation, writing meditation, asana practice, meditation questions, self-study, and studying texts. My way of working is on the one hand wildly creative and on the other hand sharply focused and disciplined.

I'd always loved astrology as a teenager. I was one of those people who always knew everyone's Sun sign and avidly read my horoscope. After a long absence, I rediscovered astrology about ten years ago while doing research for my first book, *Yoga Through the Year*. I'm not exactly sure how it happened, but somehow it just felt natural and right to focus on the zodiac signs at the same time as I was relating yoga to the seasons. By a series of happy coincidences, an old-fashioned but wonderfully wise book on astrology came into my hands, and I became fascinated by the subject once again. I felt the same frisson of excitement about astrology that I'd felt as a teenager, but this time my interest was more in the zodiac signs as twelve distinct archetypal personalities, rather than using it to predict the future or to determine individual character traits.

Has your mother or grandmother ever given you an old book of recipes handed down through the generations? There are, of course, other more modern cookbooks that you could use that are probably more efficient and up to date, but even so you love that cookbook and treasure the way it connects you to antiquated cookery lore. That's pretty much how I feel about Margaret Hone's book *The Modern Text-Book of Astrology*, which was given to me by a dear friend who is an astrologer. Although the book by modern standards is probably considered a bit quaint and old fashioned, to me it has grown to feel like a dear friend, full of magical wisdom and insight. In the same way that some people consult the tarot cards for guidance, I have used this book as a guide on my journey of interrogating the zodiac signs and relating them back to yoga.

In the book, Hone writes, "It will be found that under the headings of the names of the different planets, signs and houses comes everything which life contains, as if all were placed into their correct compartments in an enormous filing cabinet."[3] This quote certainly correlates with my own experience that all of life can be found within the wheel of the zodiac.

When I was researching my first book, I liked to work in real time, so if I was writing about and designing yoga practices for the spring equinox, I would do it around the time of the equinox. I found the same worked well for the zodiac signs, so, for example, when I was writing about and designing practices for the sign Aquarius, I would do so in the January-to-February period of the sign's dates. I found this gave me a good feel for the rhythm of the zodiac around the year.

---

3. Margaret E. Hone, *The Modern Text-Book of Astrology* (London: L. N. Fowler & Co., 1975), 19.

To start, let's look at one of the signs, Aquarius, and I'll use it to explain briefly how I go about working with a zodiac sign. As with all the signs, Aquarius has an associated planet, deity, element, color, body part, and so on. Its symbol is the water bearer and its glyph is two wavy lines, which represent waves. My first step in working with this sign, or any of the signs, would be to write down the concepts associated with it onto small squares of paper, fold them up, and literally put them into a hat. I'd then pick out about six of them, and during the month of that sign, I would focus solely on these themes. I like the idea of letting go of choice and bowing down to divine chance (other times I would use dice to help me decide on themes as well).

I know you shouldn't have favorites, but hey, Aquarius is a wonderful sign, so let's stick with it for the moment. Here's a list of themes chosen for me by the process of divine chance for Aquarius: waves, circulatory system, Uranus, the third eye, the rebel/revolution, science/detachment, the water bearer, and the Age of Aquarius. The great thing about working in this way is it leads you down avenues of exploration that you might not naturally follow. For example, during one of my Aquarius study periods, I found myself doing internet research on quantum mechanics and the wave properties of matter. I'm not someone who considers myself particularly scientifically minded, but this stuff is fascinating! Then, in order to relate the "waves" theme back to yoga, I explored wavelike breathing and integrated this into a yoga practice, including wavelike movements.

I find this way of working exciting, but I'm aware if you haven't worked like this before it could sound convoluted and complicated. And it's true that sometimes the paths I have followed on this quest have felt like a complicated maze, but fortunately the meditative process has always helped me to find a way through and out of the maze! The underlying principle of all my zodiac explorations has been to work meditatively, to listen, and to be open to guidance. Consequently, this yogic, meditative way of working has always led me from confusion to clarity, and from complication to simplicity. This in turn means that you will find clarity, simplicity, beauty, and wisdom in the Yoga by the Stars approach. I have condensed my learning from this process into nuggets of wisdom that distill the essence of each zodiac sign, and they are outlined in the zodiac chapters of this book.

You're Not the Sun Sign You Think You Are

The approach that I take to astrology in this book is to encourage you, even if only temporarily, to let go of an attachment to being defined by a specific zodiac sign (e.g., "I'm a Scorpio" or "I'm an Aquarian"). Instead, to get the most out of the book, I'd like to suggest you adopt a more open-minded, nuanced approach and recognize that you will find aspects of yourself and valuable lessons in each of the signs, regardless of whether they are *your* sign or not. If you try this, then your reward will be to find within the zodiac wheel a treasure trove of precious gems of insight, ancient wisdom, and undreamed-of opportunity.

I'm not in the business of treading on anyone's dreams, but for the purpose of this book, I do need to say a bit about precession. Due to a wobble in the Earth's rotation, the stars are in a different position, as viewed from Earth, than when the zodiac was drawn up over two thousand years ago. This means that astrology is out of alignment with the actual sky in real time.

It takes the Earth a year to complete an orbit of the Sun, and from our viewpoint here on Earth, the Sun appears to move along the ecliptic across the zodiac constellations, which means that during the cycle of a year, the Sun appears to pass across the twelve zodiac constellations. Your Sun sign, the one you read in your horoscope, is determined by the position of the Sun on the date you were born, which is why it's called a *Sun sign*. So if you were born under the sign of Virgo, the constellation Virgo was behind the Sun at the time of your birth. The Sun sign is also sometimes referred to in the popular media as the birth sign or even the star sign.

When the astrological calendar was devised over two thousand years ago, the Sun rose in Aries at the vernal equinox, whereas nowadays in the early twenty-first century the Sun rises in Pisces. In about three hundred years' time the sun will rise in Aquarius at the vernal equinox, which is why people talk about the dawning of the Age of Aquarius. Due to precession, the astrology calendar and the zodiac Sun sign dates are about a month out of synch with the location of the Sun. This means that your actual horoscope, taking precession into account, is the one ahead of the one that is assigned to you. Consequently, if you are traditionally designated Virgo, your new Sun sign, according to the actual position of the Sun, would be in Leo. (If this is news to you, sit down … take a breath … and take a few moments to readjust to this new astrological reality!)

Some astrologers argue that the effects of precession are irrelevant and their traditional systems and calculation are still valid and functional. Others suggest that the zodiac works as a system if you think of it as relating more to the season you were born in and less about the position of the Sun in your chart at the time of your birth. This argument is persuasive, as it's easy to believe that, for example, being born a Leo at the height of the summer might affect your personality and path in life differently than being born a Capricorn in the dark depths of winter. Although, it must be noted that this more seasonally oriented approach only really works for those born in the Northern Hemisphere because of the seasonal variations in the two hemispheres.

It appears that all zodiac systems, even the ones more in synch with the actual positions of celestial bodies like Vedic astrology, are by their nature intellectual constructs based on artificial, self-contained systems that are independent of external reality. However, despite this, I still find beauty and immense value from working with these systems, all of which are attempting to create a sense of order out of this vast, beautiful, disorderly universe.

Even though many of us only read our horoscope for a bit of fun, it can still be a bit disorienting when we find out that all these years, we've been reading the wrong sign! The good news is that if you are no longer defined by a specific Sun sign, this will liberate you to find the treasure in *all* the signs, not just your own.

No matter what Sun sign you are, each of the zodiac signs has the potential to bring healing and transformation into your life. If you turn back to the introduction of this book you'll find a concise guide to the healing power of each of the zodiac signs, which anyone, regardless of their sign, can use as spiritual medicine to help balance and retune their lunar and solar energies.

Let's move on now to look at some of the astrological concepts and tools that will help you to get the most out of this book and working with the wheel of the zodiac.

The Zodiac Treasure Trove

Although it might not be possible to ascertain the exact history of the origins of the zodiac, we do know that we have been bequeathed by our ancestors a zodiac treasure trove filled with celestial wisdom that we can draw upon to provide a limitless source of inspiration.

You can begin uncovering some of the treasures to be found within the wheel of the zodiac by taking a few minutes now to familiarize yourself with the following chart, which lists some of the zodiac elements that you'll come across in the book and that we'll be looking at in more detail in the rest of this chapter.

Sign	Glyph	Symbol	Ruler	Element	+ -	Color
Aries	♈	The Ram	Mars	Fire	+	Red
Taurus	♉	The Bull	Venus	Earth	-	Blues, green, pink
Gemini	♊	The Twins	Mercury	Air	+	Quicksilver
Cancer	♋	The Crab	The Moon	Water	-	Silver
Leo	♌	The Lion	The Sun	Fire	+	Gold, scarlet
Virgo	♍	The Virgin	Mercury	Earth	-	Quicksilver, gray, navy, polka dots
Libra	♎	The Scales	Venus	Air	+	Blues and pinks
Scorpio	♏	The Scorpion	Mars, Pluto	Water	-	Deep red
Sagittarius	♐	The Archer	Jupiter	Fire	+	Purple and deep blue
Capricorn	♑	The Goat	Saturn	Earth	-	Dark hues
Aquarius	♒	The Water Bearer	Saturn, Uranus	Air	+	Electric blue
Pisces	♓	The Fishes	Jupiter, Neptune	Water	-	Sea green

Zodiac Signs and Their Correspondences

Let's explore in more details now some of the elements that are found on the chart.

Zodiac Symbols and Glyphs

The Roman historian Pliny said the study of the heavens was a traditional occupation of women, who observed the seasons, drew up calendars, predicted eclipses, and performed divinations. It is thought that priestesses of the Moon goddess in Sumeria studied the constellations and identified them with various symbolic figures.[4]

The zodiac was conceived to be like a celestial zoo by our ancestors. They envisioned the zodiac constellations as animal shapes that were thought to impart the qualities of the same creatures to those humans born under the various signs: for example, a Taurean was expected to be bull-like, a Cancerian crab-like, and so on.

---

4. Barbara G. Walker, *The Woman's Dictionary of Symbols and Sacred Objects* (New York: HarperCollins Publishers, 1988), 284.

The twelve zodiac symbols, which today are not all animal symbols, can be very rewarding to work with. For example, Leo's symbol, the lion, can connect us to the exceptional capacity for cooperation displayed by lionesses or the power of the lion's roar. For the zodiac sign Cancer, there is the crab symbol. We observe how the crab withdraws back into its shell when threatened, and we can use this as a starting point to explore ideas around privacy and the public versus private, so pertinent in today's world of social media. Gemini's symbol, the twins, gives us the opportunity to focus on dualities, such as light and dark, active and passive, and so on. When we study Sagittarius, its symbol of the archer calls us to find out more about archery and to relate that to the power of intention. As you can see, it can be inspiring and fun to play around with the zodiac symbols, and then in turn we can relate our findings back to our life and our yoga practice.

Each of the twelve zodiac signs also has a pictorial symbol called a glyph. These ancient astrological symbols probably precede any known writing.[5] Their potency and power come from the wisdom and knowledge encapsulated within them. A glyph can be used as a *yantra* (a visual symbol used to aid meditation). For example, in the Aries chapter of this book, we use the Aries glyph as a yantra. When I contemplated the Aries glyph, the image that arose in my mind was of a green shoot pushing up through the soil (a sense of new growth, grounding, rebirth, and renewal), and it was this image that formed the inspiration for the Aries yoga practice.

Ruler: Planetary Influences and Archetypes

The earliest astrology-astronomy grew from our ancestors studying the heavenly bodies and connecting them with happenings on Earth. Kings, emperors, and other rulers consulted early astrologer-astronomers to predict future events, forewarn of bad omens, and find out when battles were well or poorly aspected. The study of the night sky was also essential for communities dependent on the land to garner knowledge about the weather and the changing seasons.

Although astrology and astronomy have common roots, over time, as science developed, a schism developed between them and their paths diverged. Astronomy is the study of the universe, examining the positions, motions, and properties of celestial objects, whereas astrology attempts to study how those positions, motions, and properties affect people and events here on Earth. Although the two paths might appear irreconcilable,

---

5. Hone, *The Modern Text-Book of Astrology*, 69.

many astronomers express a sense of profound gratitude to their astrological predecessors, acknowledging their indebtedness to them for the detailed records they kept of events in the night sky, some of which are still studied by astronomers today.

It's also true that some astronomers question astrology's claim that distant planetary happenings can influence human activity here on Earth. Astrologers counter this argument by noting that the Moon (which is considered a dwarf planet) does have an influence over our lives, so why not the other planets? Scientists counter this by saying that the planets are too distant to have any noticeable effect. However, I'd like to propose that whatever your position on this, there's still immense benefit to be gained from working with planetary archetypes, which contain the ancient wisdom of the myriad cultures who have projected their lives and wisdom onto the celestial canvas of the night sky. We can all recognize the planetary archetypes, with their canon of gods and goddesses, which evoke a response in us from deep within our subconscious. It can be transformational to explore these energies playing out within our own person.

Planetary archetypes, such as Mercury, the winged messenger of the gods, can be great fun to work with. In the Gemini chapter you'll find a yoga practice inspired by Mercury that uses the imagery of winged feet and a helmet to give a buoyant and uplifting effect to the practice.

Working with the planets in this way can also be thought-provoking and revealing. In the Pisces chapter we explore the planet Neptune, which is characterized by that which is veiled and hidden. Working with Neptune's energy allows us to plumb the depths of our subconscious and to uncover veiled and hidden forces at play in our lives. Once we have shone the light of day on these hidden influences, we can make conscious choices about how to work with them and so move forward with our life.

The jovial Jupiter teaches us about enjoying life and being expansive. Saturn teaches us about gravitas. Uranus evokes the wisdom of extreme old age. Pluto enables us to take advantage of sharp, sudden, eliminative energy. Mars empowers us to assert ourselves in the world. Venus enable us to appreciate beauty, uncover our hidden talents, and fulfill our potential and blossom. I hope I've whetted your appetite for the fun, insights, and transformation that can come from working with the planetary archetypes.

Element: The Zodiac and the Elements

Each zodiac sign is assigned an element: fire, earth, air, or water. This element determines the characteristics of the sign. The elements are also called the triplicities because there are three signs assigned to each of the elements.

Fire: Aries, Leo, and Sagittarius

Earth: Taurus, Virgo, and Capricorn

Air: Gemini, Libra, and Aquarius

Water: Cancer, Scorpio, and Pisces

It's interesting to note that in some Hindu systems the elements are referred to as the *tattvas*, and they are rather poetically described in this way:

- Water (*apas*) is a silver crescent moon.
- Air (*vayu*) is a blue circle.
- Fire (*tejas*) is a red triangle.
- Earth (*prithivi*) is a yellow diamond.
- The fifth element, spirit (*akasa*), is a black or indigo egg and is referred to as the void.

In this system the colors of the elements are black, white, red, yellow, and blue, which are the primary colors, and all other colors can be made from combining these colors. Likewise, the Hindus believed that from these elemental building blocks everything in the world could be created.[6]

Active and Passive Qualities of the Zodiac Signs

The signs are designated as alternately active or passive starting from Aries, which is active. The fire and air signs are active, while the earth and water signs are passive.

Active: Expressive, outgoing, extroverted, energetic, assertive, expansive, confident

Passive: Reflective, introverted, receptive, intuitive, thoughtful, contemplative

If you are familiar with the concept of yin and yang, then active corresponds with yang and passive with yin. Active is energizing and expansive like an inhalation, and

---

6. Walker, *The Woman's Dictionary of Symbols and Sacred Objects*, 106.

passive is relaxing like an exhalation. Although it's traditional to label active as "masculine" and passive as "feminine," I don't use this gendered form of categorization because I don't like the way that it reinforces limiting gender stereotypes.

When writing this book, I really enjoyed the way that the alternating active/passive designation of the signs gave each of the zodiac sign chapters in this book its own rhythm. As you read through the book, see if you can spot the active-passive pulse beating through all the chapters.

The Zodiac Wheel and the Chakras

Each zodiac sign is associated with a chakra, as shown in the following figure.

Chakra and Its Location	Sanskrit Name	Associated Color	*Bija* Mantra	Zodiac Sign
Crown Chakra *The space just above the crown of the head*	*Sahasrara*	Violet, gold, white	*Om*	Aquarius
Third Eye Chakra *Between the brows*	*Ajna*	Indigo	*Am* or *Om*	Sagittarius, Pisces
Communication Chakra *Throat*	*Vishuddha*	Blue	*Ham*	Gemini, Virgo
Heart Center Chakra *Heart*	*Anahata*	Green	*Yam*	Libra, Taurus
Solar Plexus Chakra *Upper abdomen*	*Manipura*	Yellow	*Ram*	Aries, Leo
Creation Chakra *Lower abdomen*	*Svadhisthana*	Orange	*Vam*	Cancer, Scorpio
Root Chakra *Base of the spine*	*Muladhara*	Red	*Lam*	Capricorn

The Zodiac Signs and Their Associated Chakras

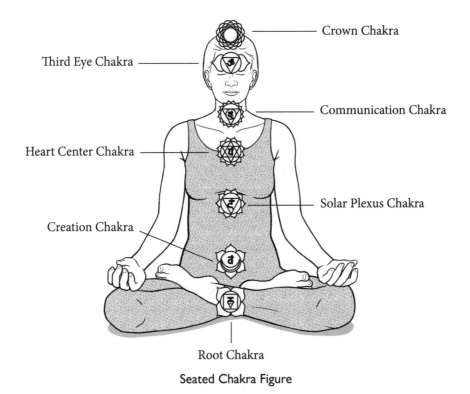

Crown Chakra

Third Eye Chakra

Communication Chakra

Heart Center Chakra

Solar Plexus Chakra

Creation Chakra

Root Chakra

Seated Chakra Figure

The Zodiac Signs and Their Associated Chakras

Both astrology and the chakra system have a poetic symbolism that we can draw from to inspire our yoga practice. Astrology teaches us the poetry of our relationship with a vast mysterious cosmos, of which we are a miniscule but important part. And inversely the chakras map out a poetic, symbolic map of our inner solar system, helping us locate the constellations of our own subtle energy system. No one can define exactly what the chakras are or where they are located, so each time you work with the chakras, you are an explorer of inner space.

It can be rewarding to work with the *bija* (seed) mantras associated with each chakra. They are so simple … and you don't even need to have a tuneful voice to join in! I've integrated the *bija* mantras into several of the zodiac-inspired yoga practices in this book. They combine well with simple yoga movements and give a meditative focus to the practice. To get a feel for working with them, try the following Chakra Seed Mantra

Meditation. In the Capricorn chapter, chapter 13, you'll find a more in-depth version of this meditation, which helps you build on the skills you've developed here.

MEDITATION

Chakra Seed Mantra

This meditation gives a simple, enjoyable way of connecting with the seven main chakras. It works well at the end of a yoga session, and it could be used to conclude any of the yoga practices in this book. The meditation helps shift stuck, stagnant energy, clearing blocked subtle energy channels and helping our energy flow more freely.

Allow 10 minutes.

In this meditation we take our awareness from the root chakra, at the base of spine, up to the crown chakra at the top of the head. We sequentially bring our awareness to, and feel into, the part of the body where the chakra is located, and then we repeat three times the *bija* mantra associated with that chakra.

If meditating lying down, we use the seed mantras silently. This is exquisitely relaxing as well as gently energizing. If done sitting, the seed mantras can be vocalized, repeated silently internally, or a combination of both. I like to vocalize the mantras from the root chakra up to the crown of the head and then repeat the mantras silently on the journey down from the crown of the head back to the root chakra at the base of the spine.

To begin, find yourself a comfortable position: either an erect sitting position or lying on the floor in Relaxation Pose (*Savasana*).

1. Bring your awareness to the base of the spine. Feel into this area and notice any sensations that are present. On the exhale, repeat the mantra *Lam* (pronounced *lum*) three times, either silently or out loud.

2. Bring your awareness to the lower abdomen. Feel into this area and notice any sensations that are present. Repeat the mantra *Vam* (pronounced *vum*) three times, either silently or out loud.

3. Bring your awareness to the upper abdomen. Feel into this area and notice any sensations that are present. Repeat the mantra *Ram* (pronounced *rum*) three times, either silently or out loud.

4. Bring your awareness to the heart center. Feel into this area and notice any sensations that are present. Repeat the mantra *Yam* (pronounced *yum*) three times, either silently or out loud.

5. Bring your awareness to the throat. Feel into this area and notice any sensations that are present. Repeat the mantra *Ham* (pronounced *hum*) three times, either silently or out loud.

6. Bring your awareness to the space between the brows. Feel into this area and notice any sensations that are present. Repeat the mantra *Om* (pronounced *aum*) three times, either silently or out loud.

7. Bring your awareness to the space just above the crown of the head. Feel into this area and notice any sensations that are present. Repeat the mantra *Om* (pronounced *aum*), three times, either silently or out loud.

Then repeat the steps above, in reverse order, from seven back to one. Observe how you are feeling having completed the meditation. Ground yourself by noticing the sensations associated with where your body is in contact with the floor or your support.

If you are lying, come back to sitting. Bring your hands together at the heart center. Make your hands and fingers into the shape of a fully open lotus flower (*Padma Mudra*). Then gently curl the fingers, so the hands look like a flower closing back to bud. As you do this, picture all your seven chakras closing back to bud too. Repeat three times, inhaling as your hand-flower opens and exhaling as it closes back to bud. This picturing of the chakras closing ensures that we are not too open after working with the chakras and that we have the necessary psychic protection in place to function well in our everyday life.

Planning Your Journey around the Wheel of the Zodiac

Now that you are familiar with the astrological approach used in this book, you're ready to dive into the rest of the book. First, I suggest that you read the next chapter, "The Sun, the Moon, Yoga, and You," as this will help you to orient yourself, ready for the zodiac sign chapters ahead. After that it's up to you where you start with the twelve zodiac sign chapters. You could either read them all through in order, or dive into whatever time of the year you are in: for example, if it's February, start with Aquarius. You might also start with your Sun sign. It's entirely up to you. The book is circular, and each chapter is a complete, independent entity, as well as being in relationship with every other chapter in the book. Remember, regardless of your sign, each of the zodiac signs has a healing potency that can be used by everyone. Trust your intuition to guide you to the chapter that will be most valuable for you.

CHAPTER 3

The Sun, the Moon, Yoga, and You

In his Yoga Sutra the ancient Indian philosopher Patanjali describes how the yogis of ancient times oriented themselves by turning their gaze up to the stars and then performing an amazing mental backflip, turning their gaze back in upon themselves and discovering contained within themselves the stars, the Sun, the Moon, and the entire universe:

> From perfect discipline of the sun, one has knowledge of the worlds.
> From perfect discipline of the moon, one has knowledge of the arrangements of the stars.
> From perfect discipline of the polestar, one has knowledge of the movements of the stars.
> From perfect discipline of the circle of the navel, one has knowledge of the body's arrangement.[7]

In the Yoga Sutra Patanjali gives a route map for the yogi that, when followed, leads from an outward solar system–wide journey of exploration, returning to an

---

7. Barbara Stoler Miller, *Yoga: Discipline of Freedom; The Yoga Sutra Attributed to Patanjali* (New York: Bantam Books, 1998), 66, sutras 3.26–3.29.

inward journey of contemplation and self-discovery. Hence, yoga teaches us to zoom our awareness out to survey this vast, mysterious universe that we inhabit and then to zoom our awareness back inward, discovering that we are one with that same cosmos. In sutra 3:33 Patanjali states, "From intuition, one knows everything."[8]

Millennia later, scientists are only just catching up with what the yogis intuited about the cosmos and our relationship to it. The ancient yogis turned their gaze inward and discovered the cosmos mirrored within their own bodies, and now scientists confirm that "most of the elements of our bodies were formed in stars over the course of billions of years and multiple star lifetimes."[9] This could explain our fascination with the stars—we are literally made of the stuff of stars.

In *Yoga: Immortality and Freedom* Mircea Eliade writes that "a considerable proportion of Indian mystical physiology is based upon the identification of 'suns' and 'moons' in the human body."[10] *Hatha yoga* is the system of uniting our sun (*ha*) and moon (*tha*) energies in the body. In other words, we find the macrocosm of the universe within the microcosm of the human body. Through the practice of yoga, you get to "see a World in a Grain of Sand" and "hold Infinity in the palm of your hand."[11]

Finding Your Place in the Cosmic Dance

Yoga isn't about finding answers to all the questions of existence; it's about learning to appreciate and fully participate in this great, mysterious cosmic dance. It's truly remarkable that thousands of years ago yogis uncovered universal, cosmological truths through intuitions revealed during meditation, as well as by looking out and observing the world around them. Like the ancient yogis, you too can hone your intuitive understanding of your place in the world through yoga and meditation, as well as by studying and discovering all you can about your world and the cosmos it turns in. The gift of yoga is that we become curious about the world and our place within it.

---

8. Stoler Miller, *Yoga*, 67.

9. Kerry Lotzof, "Are We Really Made of Stardust?" UK Natural History Museum, June 4, 2018, http://www.nhm.ac.uk/discover/are-we-really-made-of-stardust.html?gclid=EAIaIQobChMI2dif1cP_3wIVyr3tCh3x8gMAEAAYASAAEgLFGvD_BwE.

10. Mircea Eliade, *Yoga: Immortality and Freedom* (Princeton, New Jersey: Princeton University Press, 1958), 97.

11. William Blake, "Auguries of Innocence," in *Poets of the English Language* (New York: Viking Press, 1950), lines 1 and 3.

Earth is one of eight planets (and one dwarf planet, Pluto) that orbit around the Sun. It takes one year for Earth to orbit the Sun. Simultaneously our Sun and its entire solar system are orbiting the center of the Milky Way galaxy, moving at about 450,000 miles per hour in this huge orbit. The planet we call home is in an outer spiral of the Milky Way galaxy, and it takes our sun and planets approximately "230 million Earth years [a cosmic year] to make one complete orbit around the Milky Way."[12] And, if that isn't mind-boggling enough, remember that the whole galaxy is also rotating … and our sun is only one of millions of stars in the galaxy.

When we step onto our yoga mat, we are looking to find an experience of tranquil stillness in a world that is constantly on the move. Consider this: during the first few minutes of stepping onto your mat, you will have moved more than 12,500 miles (20,000 kilometers) in orbit around the galaxy's center! Bearing this in mind, is it any wonder that you sometimes feel a bit jittery at the start of your yoga practice? The extraordinary thing is that we are all space travelers, traveling on a wonky rock hurtling through space at around 500,000 miles an hour.

The Where Am I? Meditation in the Aries chapter is a good way of exploring your place in the cosmos and finding your cosmic bearings.

Sun, We Salute You!

The Sun is at the heart of our Yoga by the Stars approach. The Sun's energy gives life to Earth, and without it there would be no life on our planet. Its gravity holds everything in the solar system together. The Sun-Earth relationship is what drives the seasons, weather, climate, and ocean currents.

The symbol for the Sun is a dot within a circle. It is the primal *yantra*; simple and profound. Since ancient times the Sun symbol has been used to represent the primal womb containing the spark of creation, like the *bindu* within the *yoni yantra* of Hindu tradition.[13] It can be very rewarding to use the Sun symbol as a *yantra* (a visual aid for meditation). The Create Your Own Solar Mandala Meditation in the Leo chapter uses the Sun symbol as a starting point for meditation. We also use the Sun symbol as a *yantra* in the Leo yoga practice.

---

12. "Our Sun," NASA Science, last modified December 19, 2019, https://solarsystem.nasa.gov/solar-system/sun/in-depth/.

13. Walker, *The Woman's Dictionary of Symbols and Sacred Objects,* 15.

Sun Glyph

Try this: put your hand to your heart and say, "I am the sun at the center of my own life." How does that feel? When you find the Sun at the center of your life, you will have found the path of your natural orbit. You will feel centered and aligned with your life's purpose. This is the golden chalice that is the prize of all spiritual quests. You are what you seek. Thou art that.

The aim of the Yoga by the Stars approach is to empower you to locate the Sun at your center and to help you live authentically from that radiant, powerful center. Everything that forms part of you—your body, your mind, your emotions—is a constellation that revolves around a center. Are you the sun at the center of your own life's constellation? Or do you wander around at the periphery of your life looking for someone or something else to orbit around?

The Sun is at the center, and around the Sun are the twelve signs of the zodiac. You are the sun that shines a light into each of the twelve signs, revealing the treasure to be found within. Without you, without your sunlight, there is no life in the signs: it is you, your light, that brings them to life and lets them shine. The purpose of our pilgrimage around the zodiac wheel is to find the sun at the center of our life and to shine that light out into the world.

Sun Yoga

It can be fun to ask the Sun to guide you through a yoga practice. As you step onto your yoga mat, ask yourself, if the Sun were leading my yoga practice today, where would it take me? Then silently say to yourself: "Sun, please guide me through this yoga practice."

I find that focusing on the Sun during a yoga practice leaves me feeling happy, strong, and confident. What really impresses me is the creativity that you can tap into and harness with the Sun as a focus. I find that the moves I come up with when the Sun is my guide surprise and delight me. Anything feels possible with the Sun as your guide, and poses that you would usually find impossible are achieved fearlessly and effortlessly.

Of course, it can feel daunting to stand on your yoga mat and have no idea what shape or form your yoga practice is going to take. However, the rewards are great, so try to approach your Sun-led yoga practice with an open mind and courage; be open to suggestion; listen to your inner wisdom and let it guide you; experiment and be prepared to be surprised! Or, if you don't feel ready yet to try creating your own Sun-powered yoga practices, try the one at the end of this section.

During the process of creating the Sun Yoga Practice that follows, the idea came to me to bring my hands to my solar plexus area and to radiate like the Sun. This felt right for me, although you might get a different insight that's right for you. While holding standing poses, such as the Triangle Pose (*Trikonasana*), I focused on a warm sun at my center, radiating out. I breathed and focused on radiating sunshine. This felt healing and calming and made me happy. The insight also came to me that "correct alignment" in a pose is not imposed from the outside, but rather is a sense of rightness in the pose, felt from the inside. So the "perfect pose" is the pose that feels perfect to you, even though it might not be textbook alignment. This felt liberating!

One of the gifts that my Sun yoga experiments gave me was the inspiration for the following Sun Yoga Blessing:

Sun Yoga Blessing

I dedicate this yoga practice to the Earth, the sky, the Sun, and the Moon. Today may my feet be firmly planted on the warm earth, may my mind and heart remain open and spacious like the clear blue sky, may the warmth and healing light of the Sun invigorate and inspire my practice, may the Moon guide me to the wisdom of my own ebb and flow.

Today I especially ask for guidance from the Sun. I send thanks to this bright star at the center of my world, for giving me life and sustaining life on our planet Earth. Please inspire me with your warmth and healing light, so that in turn I may radiate that light back out into the world in a positive and loving way. Breathing in, my own inner sun is recharged and revitalized, breathing out, rays of warm healing light radiate around my body.

Today I let go of all sense of grasping in my yoga practice. I am grateful for the many blessings I receive. Please give me the patience, wisdom, and trust to stay within the circle.

And so it is by your grace.

Salute to the Sun (*Surya Namaskar*)

Next, I'll give you instructions for Salute to the Sun (*Surya Namaskar*), which is a sequence that you can either use on its own or as part of the Sun Yoga Practice that follows. Feel free to substitute your own favorite version of Salute to the Sun if you prefer. If you feel the need to warm-up to prepare for this sequence, then use the Universal Warm-Up Routine in chapter 1.

1. Mountain Pose (Tadasana) *with Sun visualization*

Stand in Mountain Pose, hands in prayer position (*Namaste*). In your mind's eye visualize the Sun rising in the sky. Now picture a warm, glowing sun at your solar plexus radiating warmth and light and keep this image in mind as you perform the Salute to the Sun.

Mountain Pose with Sun visualization

2. Mountain Pose (Tadasana) *into Standing Forward Bend* (Uttanasana)

From Mountain Pose (*Tadasana*) raise your arms out to the sides and up above your head and come down into a Standing Forward Bend (*Uttanasana*).

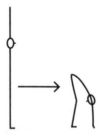

Mountain Pose into Standing Forward Bend

3. Bend knees and arch back

Bend the knees and arch the back, and then come back down into the Standing Forward Bend (*Uttanasana*).

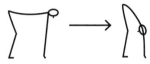

Bend knees and arch back

4. *Plank Pose* (Chaturanga Dandasana)

Step the legs back, one at a time, into Plank Pose (*Chaturanga Dandasana*), positioning the whole body in one long line.

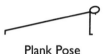

Plank Pose

5. *Plank Pose* (Chaturanga Dandasana) *into Child's Pose* (Balasana)

From Plank Pose (*Chaturanga Dandasana*), drop the knees to the floor, sitting back into Child's Pose (*Balasana*). Rest here for a few breaths.

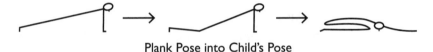

Plank Pose into Child's Pose

6. *Child's Pose* (Balasana) *into Upward-Facing Dog* (Urdhva Mukha Svanasana)

From Child's Pose (*Balasana*) come into Upward-Facing Dog (*Urdhva Mukha Svanasana*).

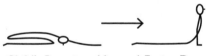

Child's Pose into Upward-Facing Dog

7. *Downward-Facing Dog Pose* (Adho Mukha Svanasana) *with Leg Lifts*

From Upward-Facing Dog (*Urdhva Mukha Svanasana*) turn your toes under and swing back into a Downward-Facing Dog Pose (*Adho Mukha Svanasana*). Stay for a few breaths in the pose. If you wish, lift one straight leg to hip height; if that feels okay, lift the leg higher so that it is in line with the torso. Do not tilt the pelvis. Repeat on the other side. Repeat 4 times each side.

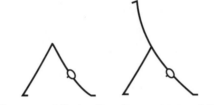

Downward-Facing Dog Pose with Leg Lifts

8. *Lunge Pose* (Anjaneyasana)

From Downward-Facing Dog Pose (*Adho Mukha Svanasana*) bring your right foot forward into Lunge Pose (*Anjaneyasana*).

Lunge Pose

9. *Standing Forward Bend* (Uttanasana) *into arched back*

Bring the other foot forward, coming into a Standing Forward Bend (*Uttanasana*). Bend the knees and arch the back.

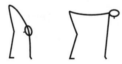

Standing Forward Bend into arched back

10. *Standing Forward Bend* (Uttanasana) *into standing*

Come back into the Standing Forward Bend (*Uttanasana*) and stay for a few breaths. Then sweep the arms out to the sides and up above the head, coming back up to standing.

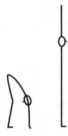

Standing Forward Bend into standing

11. *Mountain Pose* (Tadasana) *with Sun visualization*

Bring the hands back into the Prayer Position (*Namaste*) and rest here for a few breaths. As you rest, picture in your mind's eye the Sun rising in the sky. Then picture a warm, glowing sun at your solar plexus radiating warmth and light, and keep this image in mind as you perform another round of the Salute to the Sun.

Mountain Pose with Sun visualization

This Salute to the Sun can either be used on its own or integrated into another yoga practice, like the Sun yoga practice that follows.

Here is an overview of the Salute to the Sun sequence as an aide-mémoire for you:

Salute to the Sun Overview

1. Mountain Pose with Sun visualization.
2. Mountain Pose into a Standing Forward Bend.
3. Bend knees, arch back, and back into Standing Forward Bend.
4. Plank Pose.
5. Plank Pose into Child's Pose.
6. Child's Pose into Upward-Facing Dog.
7. Downward-Facing Dog with Leg Lifts × 4 on each side.
8. Lunge Pose.
9. Standing Forward Bend.
10. Standing Forward Bend to standing.
11. Mountain Pose with Sun visualization.

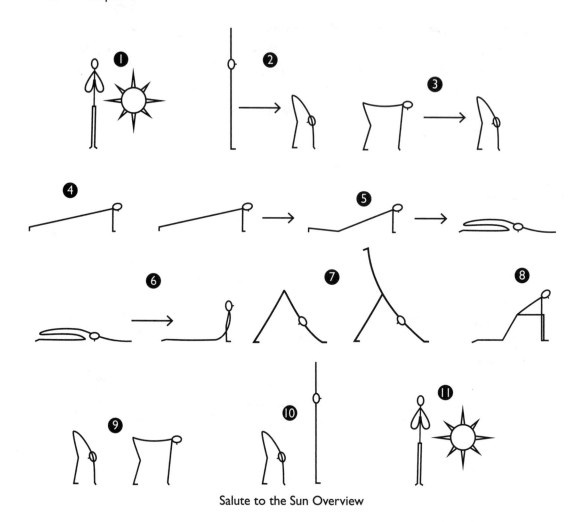

Salute to the Sun Overview

Sun Yoga Practice

In this practice we locate the Sun within our own body and picture sunlight radiating out from our center and around the body. The practice is healing, calming, strengthening. It builds confidence, lifts mood, energizes, uplifts, empowers, builds determination, expands your sense of what is possible, and strengthens intention. At the end of these instructions you'll find an illustrated aide-mémoire for the whole practice.

Allow 20 to 30 minutes.

If you feel the need to warm up to prepare for the following practice, then use the Universal Warm-Up Routine in chapter 1.

1. Mountain Pose (Tadasana) with Sun visualization

Stand in Mountain Pose (*Tadasana*), hands in prayer position (*Namaste*). In your mind's eye visualize the Sun rising in the sky. Now picture a warm, glowing sun at your solar plexus radiating warmth and light, and keep this image in mind as you perform the asanas in this practice.

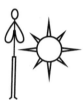

Mountain Pose with Sun visualization

2. Warrior 2 Pose (Virabhadrasana 2)

Take the legs wide apart, turning the left foot slightly in and right foot out. Bend the right knee. Take the arms out at shoulder height, palms facing down. Turn your head to look along your right arm. Stay here for a few breaths, picturing a Sun at your center radiating rays of healing light around the body. From here, before changing sides, on this same side do steps 3 and 4, Reverse Warrior Pose (*Viparita Virabhadrasana*) and Extended Side Angle Pose (*Utthita Parsvakonasana*).

Warrior 2 Pose

3. *Reverse Warrior Pose* (Viparita Virabhadrasana)

From Warrior 2 Pose (*Virabhadrasana* 2), rest your left hand on the outside of your left thigh, raise your right arm, and lean back toward the left leg. Stay a few breaths, and then go into Extended Side Angle Pose.

Reverse Warrior Pose

4. *Extended Side Angle Pose* (Utthita Parsvakonasana)

Briefly come back into Warrior 2 Pose (*Virabhadrasana* 2). From here take your right forearm to rest on your bent right knee or bring your right fingertips to rest on the floor or on your ankle. Your left hand reaches up toward the sky or over toward your ear. Keep your chest rotating skyward. Stay for a few breaths, radiating rays of warm sunlight from your center.

Repeat steps 2, 3, and 4 on the other side.

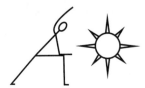

Extended Side Angle Pose

5. *Salute to the Sun* (Surya Namaskar)

You can do a few rounds of Salute to the Sun (*Surya Namaskar*) here (see page 38), or if you are pushed for time, skip this and go straight to step 6.

6. *Seated Forward Bend* (Paschimottanasana)

Sit tall with your legs outstretched (to ease the pose, bend the knees). Inhale and raise your arms. Exhale and fold forward over the legs. Inhale and return to starting position. Repeat 6 times and on the final time stay for a few breaths in the pose. As you stay in the pose, maintain a sense of sunlight radiating out from your center.

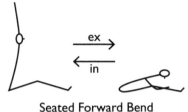

Seated Forward Bend

7a. *Bridge Pose* (Setu Bandhasana)

Lie on your back, knees bent and hip width apart and arms by your sides. Slowly peel the back from the floor and clasp the hands under the body (or, if more comfortable, leave the arms by your sides). Stay in the pose for a few breaths, visualizing a sun at your center radiating healing light. Exhale and release the clasped hands and lower the back to the floor.

7b. *Bridge Pose* (Setu Bandhasana) *with leg raise*

Come into Bridge Pose (*Setu Bandhasana*) as in step 7a. Bend one knee into the chest and then straighten the leg, heel toward the ceiling. Stay for a few breaths. Do not allow the pelvis to tilt to one side. Repeat on the other side.

To work more gently, skip step 7b, Bridge Pose with leg raise.

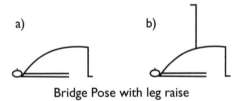

Bridge Pose with leg raise

8. *Upward-Facing Bow Pose* (Urdhva Dhanurasana)

If you are an experienced yoga practitioner, after Bridge Pose (*Setu Bandhasana*), you might want to include the advanced backbend Upward-Facing Bow Pose (*Urdhva Dhanurasana*). With the Sun as your guide, anything seems possible! I am not giving instructions for Upward-Facing Bow Pose because if you haven't done it before, it's best to learn it from a qualified yoga teacher.

If this pose isn't possible for you (like me) at present, then just rest for a few breaths with both knees bent and feet on the floor, and simply visualize yourself in the Upward-Facing Bow Pose. Or repeat Bridge Pose (7a) again.

Upward-Facing Bow Pose

9. *Knees-to-Chest Pose* (Apanasana)

Hug the knees into the chest. Rest here for a few breaths.

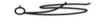

Knees-to-Chest Pose

10. *Tortoise Pose* (Kurmasana)

Sit tall, legs just over hip width apart and knees bent. Lower the torso into a forward bend. Slip both arms under the knees and behind you to rest on the lower back. For an easier alternative, catch hold of the outside of the ankles. Stay for a few breaths, focusing on where your body is supported by the earth beneath you and relaxing into that support.

To work more gently, substitute this pose with the Seated Forward Bend (step 6).

Tortoise Pose

11a. *Supine Twist* (Jathara Parivrtti)

Lie on your back, knees bent, feet together, arms out to the sides at shoulder height, and palms facing down. Bring both knees onto your chest. Exhale and lower both knees down toward the floor on the left. Inhale and return to center. Repeat 6 times on each side, alternating sides.

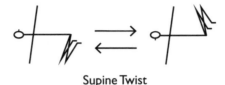

Supine Twist

11b. Supine Twist variation (Jathara Parivrtti)

Drop your knees to the left and place your left hand on your right thigh, gently persuading your legs down toward the floor. Turn your right palm up, and keeping your arm in contact with the floor, raise your arm up toward your right ear. Stay here for a few breaths, focusing on where your body is supported by the earth beneath you and relaxing into that support. Repeat on the other side.

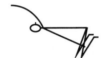

Supine Twist variation

12. Knees-to-Chest Pose (Apanasana) *into Wide Leg Stretch*

Bring the knees into the chest and rest the fingertips lightly on the knees. While inhaling, take the arms overhead and straighten the legs vertically, heels toward the ceiling. Exhale and take the legs out into a wide V shape. Inhale and bring the legs together again. Exhale and bend the knees into the chest, bringing the fingertips back to the knees. Repeat sequence 4 to 6 times.

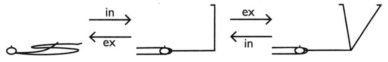

Knees-to-Chest Pose into Wide Leg Stretch

13. Relaxation Pose (Savasana) *with visualization*

Lie on your back, knees bent, feet on the floor. For comfort you could place a low cushion under your head. Visualize the Earth orbiting the Sun and the Moon orbiting the Earth. Notice any feelings this brings up for you. Then bring your awareness firmly back to Earth, as it's important to ground yourself after spending a whole practice focusing on the Sun. To do this notice where your body is in contact with the floor or your support. Allow yourself to relax down into the support of the earth beneath you. Take note of how you are feeling now after your Sun Yoga Practice. When you are ready, have a good long stretch, and slowly in your own time carry on with your day.

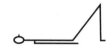

Relaxation Pose with visualization

Sun Yoga Practice Overview

   1. Mountain Pose with Sun visualization.

   2. Warrior 2 Pose.

   3. Reverse Warrior Pose.

   4. Extended Side Angle Pose. *Repeat steps 2, 3, and 4 on the other side.*

   5. Salute to the Sun (optional).

   6. Seated Forward Bend × 6.

 7a. Bridge Pose.

 7b. Bridge Pose with leg raise.

   8. Upward-Facing Bow Pose or rest a few breaths.

   9. Knees-to-Chest Pose.

 10. Tortoise Pose.

11a. Supine Twist × 6, alternating sides.

11b. Supine Twist variation. Stay a few breaths.

 12. Knees-to-Chest Pose into Wide Leg Stretch × 4–6.

 13. Relaxation Pose with visualization.

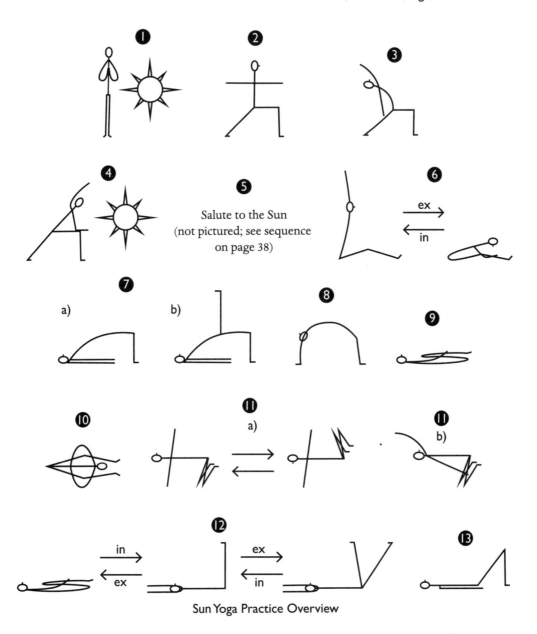

Sun Yoga Practice Overview

He-Sun, She-Moon?

Many of the older astrological texts assigned the Sun to men and the Moon to women. The Moon was said to signify the wife in a man's horoscope, while the Sun signified the husband in a woman's. Nowadays astrologers are more likely to view the Sun or Moon in a chart as reflecting the inner life of both sexes, which is more appropriate in a time when our approach to gender is more fluid and gender roles are less strictly prescribed.

I've noticed within yoga circles that it is often unquestioningly accepted that the Sun is gendered male and the Moon female. Similarly, invariably the Earth is identified as female, Mother Earth, the one who passively accepts the seed, whereas the sky and the heavens are assumed to be inherently male. It always seems odd to me that men and women who in their everyday life wouldn't dream of going along with such stereotypical projections are apparently fine with it in a yoga, "spiritual" context.

The concept of woman as yin, passive, and receptive can be traced back to Aristotle (fourth century BCE), who introduced the idea that the male seed provides the "form" of the human body. He proposed that woman's part was merely to passively receive the formative power of the male seed and so conceive a child. Ideally the baby would be male—this was considered the norm—but if things went wrong an inferior, "malformed" female would be produced. Men were perceived as fiery, hot, and active, whereas women were cold, wet, clammy, and passive. In 1827 Karl Ernst von Baer discovered the ovum, and finally it was recognized that women do have an equal share in reproduction.[14] However, many within yoga and spiritual circles still need to catch up with this shift of paradigm.

The term *Moon yoga* seems to have been adopted by the wider yoga community as a generic term for women's yoga. On one hand, of course, who wouldn't want to identify with that wonderful hazy, watery, beautiful Moon that lights up our night sky? However, on the other hand, if you are a woman, are you happy to have no light of your own and to only reflect his (the Sun's) powerful light? This assumption mirrors patriarchal society, in which his light is stronger, and she shines only by reflected glory.

There is evidence that this classification was not always so. According to Tantric scriptures, the Sun was nothing more than a garment of light for the Great Goddess.[15] There are also accounts of Sun goddesses among Eskimos and the Japanese, and the

---

14. Jean Holm, *Women in Religion,* with John Bowler (New York: Continuum, 2004), 35.

15. Walker, *The Woman's Dictionary of Symbols and Sacred* Objects, 15.

Khasis of India were accompanied by subordinate brothers who were symbolized as the moon.[16] Oriental and pre-Christian systems also frequently made the Sun a goddess.

It's interesting to note that in the tantras and yogic commentaries the right- and left-flanking subtle energy channels are often spoken of as feminine and masculine, respectively. In the *Cakrasamvara Tantra* the right channel is depicted as red tinged and white and is said to be governed by the fire element, the feminine dynamic, and the Sun. In contrast, the left channel is depicted as white tinged with red and governed by the masculine energy, the Moon, and the water elements; its vital breath is cool. These two aspects are complementary, and their union is essential in yogic practice.

The energy that resides at the crown is described as white, like brilliant crystal or diamond, and is referred to as icy cool, the Moon, and the father. Below the navel is the mother energy, which is called the Sun, and it's hot and fiery, red in color. Yogic practice joins the dualities of masculine and feminine, bringing the masculine energy of the crown of the head together with the fiery feminine energy of the lower channels. When they meet, the fiery mother melts the icy father. When the masculine and feminine are joined in the central channel, this leads to the experience of great bliss, and the yogic path is vital and complete.[17] You can explore these concepts further with the Gemini Yoga Practice and the Sun and Moon Meditation, both of which are found in the Gemini chapter, chapter 6.

I'd like to propose that if we are prepared to drop the He-Sun and She-Moon mentality, we'll all be the richer for it. Everyone benefits when our spiritual practice catches up with modern-day sensibilities that empower both sexes with the freedom to act in an authentic, life-affirming, soul-felt way. Once this happens, we are like planets that can follow the trajectory of our true orbit. Or rather, we are the Sun, shining bright and true at the center of our own solar system.

Moon, We Salute You

The Moon is the Earth's natural satellite that shines by reflecting the Sun's light. When you see moonlight reflected upon ocean, it's easy to see why in central Asia it was said that the Moon is the Goddess's mirror reflecting everything in the world, like the mirror of

---

16. Merlin Stone, *When God Was a Woman* (Orlando, FL: Harcourt Brace & Company, 1976), 2–3.

17. Judith Simmer-Brown, *Dakini's Warm Breath: The Feminine Principle in Tibetan Buddhism* (Boston, MA: Shambhala Publications, 2003), 176–78.

Maya. Persians looked upon the Moon as a mother whose love penetrated everywhere.[18] In many ancient cultures the Moon was worshipped above all other heavenly bodies, including the Sun.

The Moon speaks to us of time passing, and its waxing and waning connects us to the ebb and flow of life. The phases of the Moon teach us about the cycles of life, death, rebirth, and renewal. Out of the darkness, the New Moon arises in the night sky and speaks to us of hope reborn. The Full Moon is pregnant with possibilities. The Dark Moon reminds us to pause, rest, and recuperate.

The Earth and the Moon are in a symbiotic relationship. The gravitational pull of the Moon, and to a lesser degree the Sun, creates the ocean tides. Many people believe that the Moon's gravitational force also affects humans, as our bodies are made up of approximately 60 percent water.

Some of us notice that the phases of the Moon elicit a response in us. Of course, our response to the phases of the Moon is a very personal thing. Some of us love the flurry of energy, activity, and creativity during the waxing phase of the Moon up to when it reaches its fullness. Others prefer the more serene, contemplative, reflective energy of the waning phase of the Moon. If you regularly observe the response that the Moon's cycle elicits in you, it will help you find a rhythm of activity and rest that is uniquely healthful and energizing for you.

In ancient times calendars were based on phases of the Moon and menstrual cycles. Many women, including myself, intuitively feel that the Moon has an influence over their menstrual cycles and fertility. Although, it's interesting to note that a moonlike twenty-eight-day cycle is not necessarily the norm for most women. So it's unlikely, and possibly undesirable, that all menstruating women could simultaneously align their periods with the Moon's cycle. Anecdotally, many women notice that their best friends, flatmates, and female colleagues do seem to synch their periods. To the Greeks, *menos* meant both "moon" and "power." [19]

In astrology the key words associated with the Moon are *response* and *fluctuation*. In older texts the Sun represented spirit, the Moon represented soul, and the ascendant represented body. The Moon represents the pull of matter (subconscious), and the Sun

---

18. Barbara G. Walker, *The Woman's Encyclopedia of Myths and Secrets* (New York: HarperCollins, 1983), 670.

19. Walker, *The Woman's Encyclopedia of Myths and Secrets*, 670.

the pull of spirit (superconscious). The Moon's connection with health has always made her prominent in astrological medicine.

There are many ways you can introduce a Moon theme into your yoga practice. You can include circular sequences that mirror the phases of the Moon, such as *Chandra Namaskar* (Salute to the Moon); also see the Moonlit Tree Sequence in chapter 15, which covers Pisces. The Pisces glyph is also a great way into working with the Moon. All *pranayama* practices are a way of bringing both Sun (*ha*) and Moon (*tha*) into your practice (also see Circular Breathing in chapter 15). You could try including flowing, fluid, watery movements into your practice. We are also connecting with the ebb and flow, waxing and waning rhythm of the Moon, when we consciously attend to balancing *sthira* (effort) and *sukha* (ease) in our yoga practice. Off the mat, meditative, circular walks also have a satisfyingly Moon-like quality to them.

You could try visualizing the Moon during a yoga practice or ask the Moon to guide your intuitive practice. However, whenever you introduce a Moon focus into your yoga, it's important to remember to stay grounded. Working with a Moon theme and forgetting to ground yourself can be disorienting, so always keep an awareness of your connection with the earth beneath you and a sense of roots connecting you to the earth, giving you support and stability.

VISUALIZATION
Moon through the Trees

This visualization gives you a gentle way of working with Moon imagery. It enhances creativity and encourages illuminating inspiration. We use tree imagery and rootedness as a way of grounding ourselves and so avoiding getting "spaced out." In this way when working with Moon energies and imagery, we establish an anchor that facilitates safe space travel.

Allow approximately 10 minutes. You can use the visualization at the start or end of your yoga practice or as a stand-alone practice. It also works really well paired with the Moonlit Tree Sequence in chapter 15.

Find yourself a comfortable position, either lying down, sitting on the floor, or in a chair. Notice which parts of your body are in contact with the floor or your support; allow those parts of your body to relax down into the support of the earth beneath you.

Become aware of the natural flow of your breath. Observe the rhythm of your breathing following the full duration of each inhalation and each exhalation. At any point in this visualization it's fine to return to the anchor of observing the natural flow of the breath.

Now, imagine it's a moonlit evening and you are beside a clear, still pool. Picture a tree beside the water. Just allow the image of a tree to float into your mind. If no image comes, choose a tree that you love and feel an affinity to or one that has a quality that you would like to develop in yourself, such as the strength of the oak or the effortless surrender of the willow.

Enjoy the beauty of your tree. Picture the roots of your tree spreading deep under the soil, giving your tree strength, nourishment, and stability. The roots of the tree form a subterranean mirror image of the tree that is above the ground. Now picture the whole tree again; see its beautiful strong trunk, the pattern and texture of the bark, the branches spreading like arms and embracing the sky, and each individual leaf deep in conversation with the breeze.

Picture the landscape around your tree; fill in the details of your surroundings in a way that makes you feel grounded and earthed, safe and at home. Then, imagine that through the branches of the tree you can see a silvery white Full Moon rising in the clear evening sky. Watching the Moon makes you feel peaceful and at ease. As the Moon rises higher in the sky, you see its reflection rippling across the water. Enjoy the serene beauty of the Moon, and at the same time hold the image of the rootedness of your tree, bathed in moonlight.

When you feel ready, let go of the image of the tree and the Moon. Become aware of the natural flow of your breath. Notice the contact between your body and the earth beneath you. Imagine that like the tree, you have roots going deep down into the earth that give you strength and stability. When you are ready, begin to gently move the body, have a good stretch, and take this sense of spaciousness, lunar inspiration, and rootedness into whatever else you do today

EXERCISE

Attune to the Moon

One of the most enjoyable and accessible ways to develop and strengthen your sense of connection to the cosmos is to familiarize yourself with and attune yourself to the Moon's cycles. Compared to the other celestial bodies, the Moon is relatively close to Earth and, as has been discussed, its effect upon us is demonstrable. Whereas it's speculation whether a distant planet in your horoscope is going to have a positive or negative effect on your life, in contrast the Moon's influence is tangible.

Below is a simple guide to the phases of the Moon to watch out for:

- *New Moon:* For the first few days of the New Moon's cycle, it isn't visible in the sky. Then a waxing crescent will appear.
- *First Quarter Moon:* The waxing quarter Moon appears in the sky as a half Moon.
- *Full Moon:* The Moon has reached the height of its waxing phase and now begins to wane.
- *Last Quarter Moon:* The waning quarter Moon appears in the sky as a half Moon. After a few days, it becomes a waning crescent Moon, which soon disappears. A few days later the New Moon appears in the sky, and the lunar cycle begins over again.

You might have already noticed that your energy level and mood are affected by the phases of the Moon. You can hone this awareness by becoming consciously aware of the Moon's phase and noting its effect upon you. You can either just mentally make a note of the above or keep a written record. Approach this exercise as an experiment with an open-minded curiosity and impartiality. Let go of preconceptions and be open to learning something new. Below are four steps to help you to attune to the Moon:

1. Get the dates of the phases of the Moon onto your calendar, in your diary, on your phone, or anywhere where you can see them and be reminded of them.
2. With each phase of the Moon make a note of how you are feeling physically, mentally, and emotionally. Be aware of your energy levels, creativity, sexuality, sociability, and productivity.
3. If you have a menstrual cycle, note where you are in your cycle in relation to the phase of the Moon.
4. Notice what effect the phase of the Moon has on those close to you, your relationships, your work life, your home life, and your work-life balance.

To find out dates of the phases of the Moon, check out the Moon phase calculator on the StarDate website.[20] An online search will give you plenty of ideas for calendars, diaries, websites, and so on that will give you dates and times for the Moon phases where you are.

Take Time to Connect with the Cosmos

Whether you live in the city or the country, the sky is always there for you, and it provides the perfect way to connect with the cosmos. At any time, looking up at the sky and being mindful of it creates a sense of spaciousness and freedom. It gives us a sense of perspective, and our problems shrink back down to size. It provides a canvas for our creativity, and we find our ideas flow more freely. Gazing mindfully at the sky allows us to connect with a universe that is constantly changing. In the day you'll see clouds passing by, and at night you'll be treated to a changing starscape. It also engenders a sense of union and oneness with the world around you.

When I was a kid, I was taken on a school trip to a planetarium. My ten-year-old self was awestruck when the lights went down and the auditorium's domed ceiling morphed into a night sky twinkling with thousands of diamond-like stars. That day I learned to recognize some of the constellations. Since then, whenever I look up at the night sky, the star cluster that always seems to call out to me first is the Pleiades, also known as the Seven Sisters.

A few summers ago, I spent a couple of weeks staying in a remote cottage in rural France. When I stepped out of the house at night into the garden, there was complete darkness, no streetlights, no nearby conurbations lighting up the night sky. For a town dweller like myself, it was initially a bit scary, but mostly it was overwhelmingly beautiful as the night sky stretched out before me, "stars behind stars behind stars," as Iris Murdoch wrote, and you could clearly see the Milky Way filling up the whole sky.[21]

Ideally, if you want to stargaze, it's best to do it around the New Moon, as that's when the stars are brightest. If you're new to stargazing, check out local events where you can learn from an experienced astronomer in your community. You might also want to plan a trip to one of the many International Dark Sky Places. The Interna-

---

20. StarDate is run by the McDonald Observatory of the University of Texas at Austin. Visit the website here: https://stardate.org/nightsky/moon.

21. Iris Murdoch, *The Sea, the Sea* (London: Chatto and Windus, 1978; London: Vintage, 1999), 156.

tional Dark-Sky Association (IDA) advocates for the protection of the night sky from light pollution.[22]

Even if you live in the city and light pollution is a problem, you can still be mindful of the night sky. Mindfulness isn't about finding the ideal setting; it's about being present to what is. So even in the city, surrounded by a constellation of city lights, you can still look up at the night sky and spot faraway stars. Or take a walk under the light of the Full Moon and see moonlight dancing on the roofs of town dwellings or clouds racing across the night sky or the magic of the Moon surrounded by a rainbow halo. Taking a few minutes to mindfully look up at the sky, day or night, helps us get out of our head and to connect with this magical, mysterious, mystical cosmos that we are part of.

EXERCISE
Mindfulness of the Night Sky

Our ancestors looked up at the stars and saw them as sacred. They perceived divinity within the stars and felt that same spark of divinity within themselves. To them, the cosmos was a soulful place that they were part of and at one with. You can engender that same sense of reverence and wonder by regularly taking time to be mindful of the night sky.

Take a few minutes each day to mindfully connect with the night sky. This can be as simple as looking up at the sky out of your window or stopping your car (when it's safe to do so) and parking somewhere to look up at the sky.

A great way to promote a good night's sleep is to take a mindful walk an hour or so before bedtime. This is an enjoyable exercise to do with a companion. Every so often stop and look up at the sky. What do you see? Some nights you will see a splendid Moon; other nights it will be cloudy and no stars in sight; and on a clear night the stars will stretch out before you.

Mindfulness teaches us to use our senses and be present to what is, rather than what we would like to be. So notice what you can see, what you can hear. Notice the stream of thoughts passing through your mind. Be aware of judgments you are making and see if you can just come back to what is there before you. Take a mindful breath in, take a mindful breath out.

---

22. Visit the IDA's website for details of how to find a dark place near you: https://www.darksky.org /planning-your-next-trip-to-the-dark-side/.

If you are knowledgeable about the night sky, it can be fun to spot the various constellations. Although from a mindfulness point of view, it's also interesting to let go of that knowledge and to just look at the sky afresh with new eyes each time. The difficulty when we "know" something is that we have the tendency to categorize it and then move on without really looking. In mindfulness we are cultivating curiosity and a beginner's mind.

As well as observing the sky, you are also observing yourself. So if you feel disappointed because it's cloudy and you'd anticipated a spectacular show of shooting stars, then acknowledge those feelings with compassion and understanding. Stay mindful of bodily sensations, feeling yourself rooted to and supported by the earth beneath you. If you are walking, be aware of the contact your feet are making with the earth, with each step you take. And stay present to your breathing.

PART 2

Yoga and
the Zodiac Signs

CHAPTER 4

Empower Your Inner Warrior

Aries

March 20–April 19

Reconnect with your courageous and confident self.

If you are looking for a quiet life, yoga probably isn't for you. Yoga will tug at your sleeve and urge you to speak out when you are faced with injustice. It will help you set boundaries. If you are a habitual people-pleaser who always says yes to everyone, yoga will prompt you to say no and sound like you mean it. If you are someone who's scared of life, yoga will take you by the hand and say, "Yes, we can do this!" Yoga won't give you a quiet life, but it will fire you up and make life come alive again. It will be a life worth fighting for.

Yoga helps us harness that same growing energy that prompts a plant to push green shoots up through the soil in spring. Through our yoga practice, we are reborn. Once again, we experience newness, freshness, excitement, and childlike innocence. This is the beginner's mind; our newfound curiosity pushes us to grow toward the light. We step out into the sunshine. Like a spring flower, we turn our face to the Sun and are inspired to grow and develop. As we unfurl, there may be growing pains, but like a seed in the soil, we are supported by the earth, and we know we stand on solid ground.

We breathe in and we are inspired. We are energized by our inhalation and we push forward toward our goals. Our exhalation helps us remove any obstacles that stand in the way of realizing our dreams. We know when to push and when to yield. Our practice of yoga endows us with the strength to push hard when the time is right.

Kali Ma, the Hindu triple goddess of creation, preservation, and destruction, sometimes manifests as Durga, a warrior queen who "personified the fighting spirit of a mother protecting her young."[23] Yoga puts fire in your belly. It ignites a creative spark within. We are fired up and we live our life with passion. We love, we care, and we are prepared to fight for what we believe in. We are spiritual warriors, both on and off the mat.

The Bhagavad Gita, the best known of all the Hindu scriptures, teaches that if we wish to find the peace of yoga, we must be prepared to fight the battle of life. Some things are worth fighting for, and yoga is one of them. Your first warrior act might be to fight for the time and space to practice. To defend your right to take some time for yourself. To fiercely guard that precious time.

Yoga perhaps conjures up an image for you of relaxation and escapism. Yoga isn't simply an abstract concept of "love"; it is also a force that inspires you to stand up and fight for what you believe in. It gives you the strength to persist, the armor to protect you from life's blows, and the inner wisdom of the warrior.

Yoga Inspired by Aries

Aries is ruled by the warlike planet Mars. Its element is fire and its color red. In the Aries-inspired yoga practice that follows, we use poses such as the Warrior Pose (*Virabhadrasana*) to build up strength and courage. We fire up our intentions by chanting the seed mantra *Ram*, associated with the solar plexus chakra (*manipura*), and the development of personal power. At the same time as we fire up our courage, we also connect to our loving self with the affirmation *I am filled with love and courage*.

The parts of the body associated with Aries are the head and the adrenals. The mental energy required to assert ourselves and take action can lead to restless, agitated states of mind, with adrenaline pumping through our system. It's the same energy we see in the headstrong ram of Aries. Our challenge is to use this surge of energy to achieve our

---

23. Walker, *The Woman's Encyclopedia of Myths and Secrets*, 258.

goals while at the same time not getting swept away or overwhelmed by it. The Aries-inspired yoga practice will help you ride this wave of energy; calm a restless, overactive mind; and stay grounded and connected to the earth beneath your feet.

For astrologers the cycle of the twelve signs of the zodiac begins with 0-degree Aries. It is the ignition key of the year. In the Northern Hemisphere it corresponds with the beginning of spring. The Aries glyph represents the ram's horns. Traditionally ram's horns were used to blow away the old year to make room for the new. This is a time of new beginnings.

In this practice we use the Aries glyph as a *yantra* (a visual symbol to aid meditation), and the inspiration for the yoga practice came from meditating on the glyph. When contemplating the Aries glyph, the image that arose in my mind was of a new, green shoot pushing up through the soil in springtime—a sense of new growth, green shoots, grounding, rebirth, and renewal. I also intuited that the glyph has the energetic quality of a fountain of water spurting up from the soil. This gave me the idea to introduce into the yoga practice a sense of springing up but also one of staying grounded, because in order to grow and expand into space, you must be rooted in the earth. In the practice, I thought it was fun to include Boat Pose (*Navasana*), which makes a similar shape to the Aries glyph and has that same sort of energy that springs up from a grounded base.

Aries-Inspired Yoga Practice

The Aries-inspired yoga practice is for everyone, not just for those born under the Aries sign. You can use the yoga practice anytime you want to build up confidence, courage, and inner strength. It will connect you to your fiery, assertive self, while at the same time helping you get in touch with a loving heart. It is energizing, revitalizing, and grounding and creates stability.

The affirmation we use in the practice is *I am filled with love and courage.* It can be shortened and coordinated with the breath:

Inhale: Love

Exhale: Courage

Allow 20 to 30 minutes.

1. *Mountain Pose* (Tadasana)

Stand tall, feet parallel and about hip width apart. Be aware of the contact between your feet and the earth beneath you. Imagine a string attached to the crown of your head, gently pulling you skyward; simultaneously let your tailbone drop and feel your heels rooting down into the earth. Now, in your mind's eye visualize the Aries glyph. Simply picture the glyph and observe whatever thoughts and feelings arise in response to this image. Carry the image of the Aries glyph into the rest of the practice.

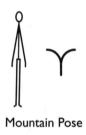

Mountain Pose

2. *Individual knee to chest warm-up*

From the Mountain Pose (*Tadasana*) raise your arms up above your head. Exhaling, draw one knee into your chest and hug it. Inhale and lower the foot back to the floor, raising arms above the head again. Repeat on the other side. Repeat 10 times, alternating sides.

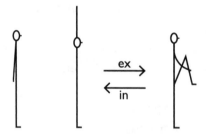

Individual knee to chest warm-up

3. *Warrior 1 Pose* (Virabhadrasana 1)

Stand tall, feet hip width apart. Turn your right foot out slightly and take a big step forward with your left foot. Inhaling, raise both arms above your head, bending the front knee over the ankle; exhaling, lower the arms and straighten the leg. Do 6 repetitions on this side, and on the final time stay for a few breaths with the arms raised. Then repeat on the other side. You can coordinate the breath and movement with the affirmation. Inhale and affirm, *Love*. Exhale, *Courage*.

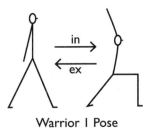

Warrior I Pose

4. *Warrior 3 Pose* (Virabhadrasana 3)

Stand tall, feet hip width apart and both arms above your head. Exhale as you tip your upper body forward, at the same time raising one straight leg behind you in line with your torso and keeping your raised arms in line with your ears (forming a human T shape). Inhale and return to starting position. Repeat 4 times and on the final time hold the pose for a few breaths. Repeat on the other side.

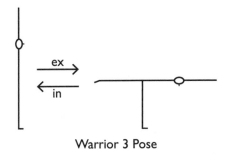

Warrior 3 Pose

5. *Warrior Pose* (Virabhadrasana) *variation into Intense Side Stretch Pose* (Parsvottanasana) *variation*

Stand tall, feet hip width apart. Step one foot forward. Inhaling, take the arms up above the head and slightly bend the front knee. Exhale and bend forward over the front leg, sweeping both arms behind the back. Inhale and come back up, arms overhead. Repeat 4 times. On the final time on this side, and before you do the other side, place both hands on the floor on either side of the front foot and step back into Downward-Facing Dog Pose (*Adho Mukha Svanasana*).

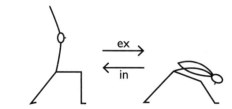

Warrior Pose variation into Intense Side Stretch Pose

6. *Downward-Facing Dog Pose* (Adho Mukha Svanasana) *into Standing Forward Bend* (Uttanasana)

Stay for a few breaths in Downward-Facing Dog Pose (*Adho Mukha Svanasana*) and then walk the hands back toward the feet. Come into a Standing Forward Bend (*Uttanasana*) and stay here for a few breaths. To ease the pose, bend the knees. Slowly uncurl, coming back up to Mountain Pose (*Tadasana*).

Repeat steps 5 and 6 on the other side.

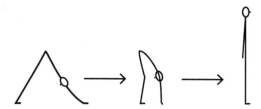

Downward-Facing Dog Pose into Standing Forward Bend

7. *Child's Pose* (Balasana) *into Upward-Facing Dog Pose* (Urdhva Mukha Svanasana)

From sitting kneeling, sit back into Child's Pose (*Balasana*), arms outstretched along the floor. Inhale, moving forward into Upward-Facing Dog (*Urdhva Mukha Svanasana*), arching your back and keeping your knees on the floor. Exhale back into Child's Pose. You can silently coordinate the breath with the affirmation. Inhale: *Love* Exhale: *Courage*. Repeat 6 times, as you move between the two poses.

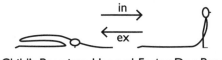

Child's Pose into Upward-Facing Dog Pose

8. *Boat Pose* (Navasana)

Come to sitting, with legs outstretched in front of you, knees bent, heels resting on the floor. Lean slightly backward, keeping a long back, with your head and neck in line with the spine and your lower abs gently pulling back toward the spine. Lift the heels from the floor and raise the legs to make a V shape out of your body (the same shape as the Aries glyph). For an easier pose keep the legs slightly bent. For more of a challenge straighten the legs. Do not round the back. As you hold the pose, silently repeat this affirmation: *I am filled with love and courage.*

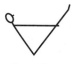

Boat Pose

9. *Seated Forward Bend* (Paschimottanasana) *and mantra* Ram

Sit tall, legs outstretched (bend the knees to ease the pose). Bring your awareness to the solar plexus. Picture a warm, radiant sun there. Inhale and raise arms. Keeping your awareness at the solar plexus, exhale and chant the mantra *Ram* (pronounced *rum*). At the end of the exhale, as you complete the chant, fold forward over the legs. Inhale and return to starting position. Repeat 6 times and on the final time stay for a few breaths in the Seated Forward Bend. Note: never strain with the breathing. Take extra breaths if you need to.

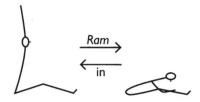

Seated Forward Bend and mantra *Ram*

10a. Bridge Pose (Setu Bandhasana)

Lie on your back; knees bent and hip width apart, arms by your sides. Slowly peel the back from the floor, clasping the hands under the body, and stay in the pose for a few breaths. To ease the shoulders, just leave your arms by your sides, palms facing down.

Bridge Pose

10b. Bridge Pose (Setu Bandhasana) *with leg raise*

Come into Bridge Pose (*Setu Bandhasana*) as in step 10a. Bend one knee into the chest and then straighten the leg, heel toward the ceiling. Stay for a few breaths. Do not allow the pelvis to tilt to one side. Repeat on the other side.

To work more gently, skip 10b.

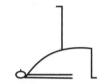

Bridge Pose with leg raise

11. Knees-to-Chest Pose (Apanasana) *into Wide Leg Stretch into Curl-Up*

Bring the knees into the chest. Rest the fingertips lightly on the knees. Inhaling, take the arms overhead and straighten the legs up to the vertical, heels toward the ceiling. Exhale and take the legs out into a wide V shape. Take an extra breath, and then on an exhale bend the knees into the chest and curl the head and shoulders from the floor into a curl-up. Still on the exhale (or take an extra breath), return to the starting position, lowering the head and shoulders back to the floor. Repeat sequence 4 to 6 times.

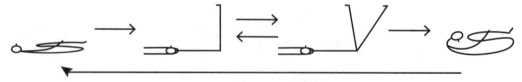

Knees-to-Chest-Pose into Wide Leg Stretch into Curl-Up

12. *Relaxation Pose* (Savasana)

Spend a few minutes relaxing, either lying down or in a comfortable sitting position. As you rest, bring back to mind a picture of the Aries glyph. What images, thoughts, and feelings does it conjure up for you? What wisdom and insight can you take from it? You don't need to strive for answers; just allow answers to arise from your subconscious in their own time. If your mind wanders, gently bring it back to visualizing the glyph. When you feel ready, let go of picturing it. Notice how you are feeling now after your Aries-inspired yoga practice. Have a good stretch, and when you are ready, carry on with your day.

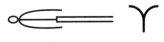

Relaxation Pose

Aries-Inspired Yoga Practice Overview

1. Mountain Pose. Visualize the Aries glyph.

2. Individual knee to chest warm-up × 10, alternating sides.

3. Warrior 1. Coordinate breath with affirmation. Inhale: *Love.* Exhale: *Courage.* Repeat × 6. On final time stay a few breaths. Repeat on other side.

4. Warrior 3 × 4. On final time hold for a few breaths. Repeat on other side.

5. Warrior variation into Intense Side Stretch Pose variation × 4 (one side only).

6. Stay a few breaths in Downward-Facing Dog Pose, and then come into Standing Forward Bend. Stay for a few breaths. Come up to Mountain Pose. Repeat steps 5 and 6 on the other side.

7. Child's Pose into Upward-Facing Dog. Inhale: *Love.* Exhale: *Courage.* Repeat × 6 as you move between the two poses.

8. Boat Pose. Hold pose and silently repeat affirmation: *I am filled with love and courage.*

9. Seated Forward Bend and mantra *Ram.* Repeat × 6, and on final time stay a few breaths in the pose.

10a. Bridge Pose. Stay in pose a few breaths.

10b. Bridge Pose with leg raise. Stay a few breaths. Repeat on other side. *For a gentler practice, skip 10b.*

11. Knees-to-Chest Pose into Wide Leg Stretch into Curl-Up. Repeat sequence ×
4–6.

12. Relaxation Pose. Spend a few minutes relaxing, picturing the Aries glyph.

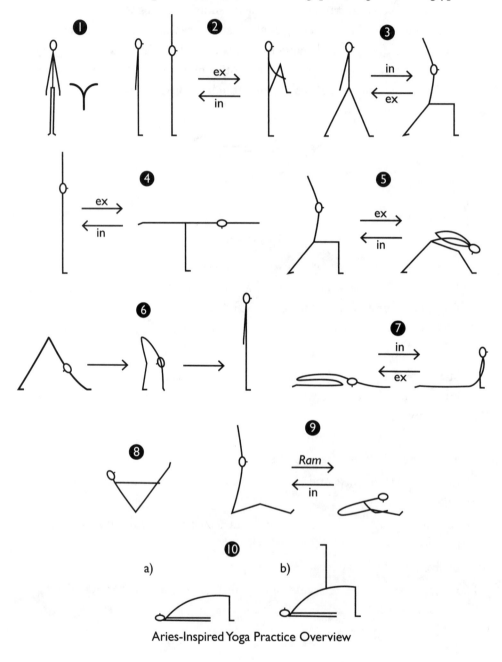

Aries-Inspired Yoga Practice Overview

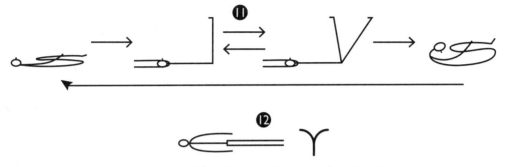

Aries-Inspired Yoga Practice Overview (continued)

MEDITATION
Where Am I?

This meditation is a valuable exercise to do at any time of the year and is relevant to all the signs. However, I have chosen to include it in the Aries chapter because it fits in with the courage and adventurousness of the sign, while at the same time teaching the skill of staying grounded and connected to the world around you.

The idea for this meditation came from looking at a picture of our galaxy in a children's book. The galaxy was depicted as a milky white swirling spiral, made up of millions of stars, against the backdrop of a night-blue sky. Helpfully, a red cross marked our place in the galaxy with the words *You are here.*

In this meditation, we ask ourselves the question "Where am I?" The question that is more commonly asked by yogis is "Who am I?" The spiritual quest of finding out who you are encourages drawing inward to discover the essence of who you are. This quest of finding oneself can in some cases lead to enlightenment; however, it can also lead to self-absorption and a disconnection from the outside world. In contrast the question "Where am I?" brings you back into your body and simultaneously unites you with the world that you are part of.

This meditation helps you gain a sense of perspective and rise above everyday concerns and preoccupations. It is elevating, engendering feelings of spaciousness and freedom. In a world that is constantly turning, this meditation teaches you how to maintain stability and stay grounded in the face of perpetual change.

Allow 15 to 20 minutes.

Find yourself a comfortable sitting position, sitting either cross-legged on the floor or in a straight-back chair. If sitting is not comfortable for you, lie down with your knees bent and feet on the floor.

Draw an imaginary circle of light around yourself. If it feels right, silently say, *I surround myself with love and light, and I am safe.*

Notice where your body is in contact with the floor or your chair. Throughout this meditation keep coming back to this sense of being connected to, and supported by, the earth beneath you.

Become aware of the natural flow of your breath. Notice the gentle sound of the breath. Throughout the meditation, keep coming back to the sounds around you and the gentle wavelike sound of the breath.

When you feel grounded and settled, ask yourself this question: *Where am I?* Repeat this question a few times, and then answer: *I am here.*

Be aware of your body. How does it feel to be here inhabiting this body? Get a sense of being fully present in your body. Become aware of the space around your body. *Where am I? I am here in my body.*

Notice the sounds inside the room and the sounds outside of the room. In your mind's eye build a picture of the room (or your immediate surroundings). *Where am I? I am here in this room (or wherever you happen to be).*

Now expand your awareness outside the room to the building you are in, to the land surrounding it, to the adjoining buildings and landscape. Picture your neighborhood, noticing landmarks such as trees, rivers, hills, or anything that is significant to you.

At regular intervals come back to a sense of being connected to, and supported by, the earth beneath you. Come back to the sounds around you and the sound of the breath. *Where am I? I am here.*

Now imagine that you have a bird's-eye view of your neighborhood. Picture what it would look like if you were looking down on your locality from above.

Then zoom out further; imagine that you are looking down on planet Earth from space. What does the blue planet look like from this viewpoint? How do you feel about the Earth looking at it from this angle? Keep a gentle, background awareness of the sound of your breath and the support of the earth beneath you.

Now expand your consciousness even further. Picture the Earth as one of eight planets orbiting the Sun. Allow yourself to consider that the Sun is one of a billion stars just in our galaxy alone.[24]

Now it's time to begin your descent back down to Earth. Picture the Earth from space. Then zoom in to your locality. Bring your awareness back to the room. Be aware of your immediate surroundings. Notice the sounds within the room, and outside the room. Notice the gentle wavelike sound of your breath. Feel the sensations associated with where your body is in contact with the floor or your support. Feel yourself held and supported by the earth beneath you. Spend a few minutes here grounding yourself and bringing yourself back to earth.

To conclude the meditation, come to a sitting position, and rest your hands on your belly. Notice the gentle rise and fall of the belly with each in- and out-breath. Then with each out-breath, silently repeat the mantra *Lam* (pronounced *lum*). This is the *bija* (seed) mantra associated with the base chakra (*muladhara*), and it is very grounding. After a few silent repetitions, begin to sound the *Lam* mantra on each exhale. With each repetition of the mantra bring your awareness down to the belly and the lower half of the body. After a few repetitions, let go of chanting.

Spend a few more minutes here, quietly observing your breath and noticing the contact between your body and the earth. Notice how you are feeling and any insights you might have gained from doing the Where Am I? Meditation. If you wish, you can write down your observations. When you are ready, carry on with your day.

Aries-Inspired Meditation Questions

See chapter 1 for guidance on how to use meditation questions. The Aries meditation theme is connecting with your inner warrior.

- What qualities would I possess if I were a spiritual warrior?
- What do I consider worth fighting for in my life?
- Which yoga poses help me build courage?

---

24. "Our Sun," NASA Science, last modified December 19, 2019, https://solarsystem.nasa.gov/solar-system/sun/in-depth/.

- How might my meditation practice assist me in developing the qualities that would help me live more courageously?
- How would my life be different if I were able to say no and mean it?
- What would I like to welcome into my life and say yes to?
- What signs are there of new green shoots appearing in my life?

CHAPTER 5

Fulfill Your Potential

Taurus

April 19–May 20

Reconnect with your passionate, sensual self and blossom!

Like blossoms on a cherry tree in spring, yoga opens you up to the beauty of your own soul. Petal by petal, it unfolds you, until you bloom into your full potential. Blossoming: you are unique, there is only one you in all of time, and you were born to blossom and to bear fruit.

Yoga brings color into a monochrome world. The world was never monochrome—it's just that you were on autopilot and didn't see the rainbow of colors. Yoga wakes you up to the beauty within and around you.

The yoga asanas, breathing practices, relaxation, and meditation open what has been closed, release what has been stuck, free what has been trapped, and unfurl those tight knots of tension. That which was hidden in darkness is brought out into the light.

Before you discovered yoga, your body was like a tightly clenched fist. Yoga uncurls your fingers and the flower of your hand blossoms. Breathe out constriction, breathe in freedom. Bend the spine forward, backward, and to the sides. Twist. The spine comes alive again; you are connected to the earth below and heaven above, rooted in the earth and open to the sky. Feet on the ground and spirit soaring.

Yoga heals you and makes you whole. The out-breath unblocks stuck energy. Breathe out, surrender, let go, and once again your energy begins to flow. Open, surrender, relax, receive, let go, yield, unfold, simply be. Welcome unity, connection, expression, sensuality, pleasure, love, and passion. The life force can move freely now and inspire you.

There is so much more to you than meets the eye. You have so much to give. Yoga is the sun that opens your flower. Once you have let go of all that unnecessary tension, what treasure trove of creativity will you discover within yourself? What hidden talents and untapped resources will you find?

Yoga opens you up to spirit, soul, love, life, living, passion, and giving. Give away what has been given to you, use yourself up, share your beauty with the world. The lotus flower is rooted in mud; it does not grow on marble.

On one level yoga practice results in a very real physical flowering; on another level there occurs a subtler flowering of awareness. Along the midline of the body, from the base of the spine to the crown of the head, are seven subtle energy centers (chakras). Traditionally, these energy centers are depicted as lotus flowers. The crown chakra is depicted as a thousand-petalled lotus, and when this opens, it results in ecstatic, blissful states of self-realization.

Yoga Inspired by Taurus

Greek, Persian, Sanskrit, and Babylonian astrologers agreed that the star group known as Taurus was a bull.[25] It was traditionally ruled by the planet Venus and the element earth. Venus is the goddess of beauty and love. Key words are *harmony*, *unison*, and *relatedness*.

When I designed the zodiac-inspired yoga practices, I did so in the month of the sign. This Taurus-inspired yoga practice evolved over a few years during the months of April and May, when all the trees are coming into blossom here in the United Kingdom. Above all, the image I held in my mind when I was designing this practice was that of a tree in blossom. Venus is associated with the period of adolescence, so the image of blossoming, with the underlying idea of opening like blossom and fulfilling potential, seemed appropriate.

---

25. Walker, *The Woman's Dictionary of Symbols and Sacred Objects*, 295.

The other Taurus-inspired ideas I held in my mind were a bull; Venus; copper (metal of Venus); blue, pink, and green (Taurus colors); the throat chakra (body part of Taurus); and the element earth. In the practice we chant the *bija* mantra *Yam* (pronounced *yum*), which is associated with the heart chakra (*anahata*) and Venus.

The tree in blossom image may at first glance seem a long way away from the traditional symbol of Taurus as the bull. However, the stability and earthiness of the sign is captured in the rootedness of the tree. The rulership of Venus is captured in the sattvic beauty of the blossom, against the backdrop of clear, blue sky. When I was designing the practice, I found myself playing around with movements that reached down to the earth and then stretched up to the sky: drawing energy up from the earth and blossoming into the sky. Pulling energy down from the sky and rooting down into earth.

Using these earth and sky images imbued me with a sense of confidence and stability, so much so that I ended up finding myself doing poses that I usually considered to be beyond my capability, such as the Crane Pose (*Bakasana*). Although I haven't included the Crane Pose in the Taurus practice below, you also may find that the practice inspires you to attempt a pose that has previously eluded you. Let your intuition guide your movements.

At the end of the Taurus-inspired yoga practice we use the mantra *Om mani padme hum,* plus the lotus flower visualization, to encourage a sense of spiritual blossoming.

Taurus-Inspired Yoga Practice

The Taurus-inspired yoga practice is for everyone, not just for those born under the zodiac sign Taurus. It will put you in touch with your sensual side and help you develop a sense of connection with the natural world. It frees blocked energy and is calming and steadying. It boosts energy and vitality and awakens creative potential.

The affirmation we use in the practice is *Love blossoms with each breath.* It can be shortened and coordinated with the breath:

Inhale: Love blossoms

Exhale: With each breath

Allow 20 to 30 minutes.

1. *Easy Pose* (Sukhasana) *with hands in Prayer Position* (Namaste)

Find yourself a comfortable seated position. Bring your hands together as if in prayer. Imagine that in the space between your two palms you are holding a sprig of a beautiful blossom. Silently repeat the affirmation: *Love blossoms with each breath.*

Easy Pose with hands in Prayer Position

2. *Cat Pose* (Marjaryasana) *into Cow Pose* (Bitilasana)

Come onto all fours. Exhale and round the back up like an angry cat. Inhale into Cow Pose (*Bitilasana*), arching the back, lifting the chest up and away from the belly, and looking slightly up. Alternate between these two positions, rounding and arching the back, and repeat 8 times. (If you have a back problem, don't arch the back.)

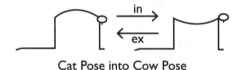

Cat Pose into Cow Pose

3. *Wave to the Moon Pose*

Start on all fours. Exhaling, thread your left arm under the torso; the back of your left hand brushes the floor. Inhaling, take the arm out to the side and up, and look up at the raised arm. Repeat 6 times, and then repeat on the other side.

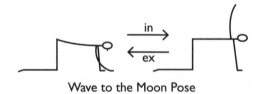

Wave to the Moon Pose

4. *Heart Chakra Sequence*

Start in Child's Pose (*Balasana*), with forearms and hands on the floor, just above your head. Inhale and come up to tall kneeling, taking your arms above your head. Exhale, chanting the mantra *Yam* (pronounced *yum*), as you cross your hands and place them at your heart. Inhale, raising the arms above your head again. Exhale, coming back to Child's Pose. Repeat the sequence 6 times.

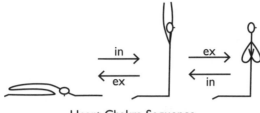

Heart Chakra Sequence

5. *Lunge Pose* (Anjaneyasana) *with arm movements*

Come to tall kneeling. Take your right foot forward; bend the knee, bringing the knee over the ankle. Rest your fingertips lightly on the tips of your ears, elbows pulled out to the side. Exhaling, round the back forward and bring the elbows to point to the front and down. Inhaling, open the elbows and lift the chest. Repeat 4 times and then stay in the open-chest position for a few breaths. Repeat on the other side.

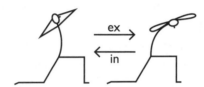

Lunge Pose with arm movements

6. *Downward-Facing Dog Pose* (Adho Mukha Svanasana)
into Standing Forward Bend (Uttanasana)

From the Lunge Pose, come onto all fours, turn the toes under, and come into Downward-Facing Dog Pose. Stay here for a few breaths, and then walk the hands backward to the feet, coming into a Standing Forward Bend. Stay here for a few breaths. To ease the pose, bend the knees more. Slowly uncurl, coming back up to standing.

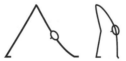

Downward-Facing Dog Pose into Standing Forward Bend

7. Standing like a tree in blossom

Stand tall like a tree. Your feet are parallel and about hip width apart, knees soft, face relaxed, and shoulders down away from the ears. Your tailbone feels heavy as though it is weighted, and the crown of your head feels light and floats skyward. Now picture the beauty of a tree in blossom. Notice its shape, the blossom's color, its fragrance. Stay here for a few breaths, enjoying the beauty of the image of the tree. Silently repeat this affirmation: *Love blossoms with each breath.*

Standing like a tree in blossom

8. Tree Pose (Vrksasana)

Stand tall, feet hip width apart, hands in Prayer Position (*Namaste*). Picture the beauty of a tree in blossom. Imagine that like a tree you have roots going from the soles of your feet way down into the earth. Then bring the sole of your right foot to rest on your inner left thigh, rotating your right knee out to the side. Either keep your hands at the heart or take your arms above the head, hands in Prayer Position. Fix your gaze on a point that is not moving. Stay for a few breaths. Repeat on the other side.

For balance problems, instead of bringing the foot onto the thigh, just rest the sole of the foot on the opposite inside ankle, or be near a wall for support.

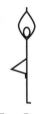

Tree Pose

9. Blossom Petal Sequence

Begin the sequence in a Standing Forward Bend (*Uttanasana*) with soft knees, and become aware of your breathing. Exhale and uncurl, slowly coming back up to standing, and imagine that as you do so, your hands are drawing energy up from the earth and through the center of the body. Bring your hands into the Prayer Position (*Namaste*), and then take the arms up above your head, shoulder width apart. As you lower the arms out to the sides, picture that you are scattering blossom petals at the same time as lowering back down into a Standing Forward Bend. Repeat a few more times, moving in a smooth, flowing, circular fashion; pulling energy up from the earth; and giving back that energy to the earth as you scatter petals.

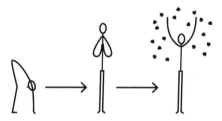

Blossom Petal Sequence

10. Lunge Pose with Twist (Anjaneyasana *variation*)

Come to tall kneeling. Take your right foot forward; bend the knee, bringing the knee over the ankle. Lean forward placing one hand on either side of the front foot. Come up onto your fingertips extending through the entire length of the spine. Do not round the upper back. Exhaling, raise your right arm out to the side and above the head, twisting your upper torso to the right and looking up at your raised hand. Inhale and return the fingertips back to the floor. Repeat the arm movement on this side 4 times. Repeat on the other side.

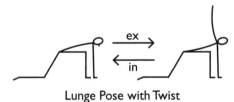

Lunge Pose with Twist

11. Child's Pose (Balasana) *into Upward-Facing Dog* (Urdhva Mukha Svanasana)

Come to kneeling and sit back into Child's Pose (*Balasana*), arms outstretched along the floor. From Child's Pose inhale and move forward into Upward-Facing Dog (*Urdhva Mukha Svanasana*), arching your back and keeping your knees on the floor. Exhale back into Child's Pose. You can silently coordinate the breath and movement with the affirmation. Inhale and affirm, *Love blossoms.* Exhale and affirm, *With each breath.* Repeat 6 times, moving between the two poses.

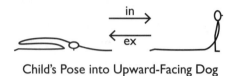

Child's Pose into Upward-Facing Dog

12. *Seated Forward Bend* (Paschimottanasana)

Sit tall, legs outstretched (bend the knees to ease the pose). Inhale and raise your arms. Exhale and fold forward over the legs. Inhale and return to starting position. You can silently coordinate the breath and movement with the affirmation. Inhale and affirm, *Love blossoms.* Exhale and affirm, *With each breath.* Repeat 6 times, and on the final time stay for a few breaths in the pose.

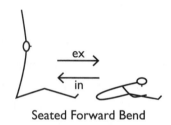

Seated Forward Bend

13. *Supine Butterfly Pose with arm movements* (Supta Baddha Konasana variation)

Lie on your back, with your knees spread out to the sides, soles of the feet together, and hands resting on your belly or the tops of the thighs. For comfort, prop your knees on bolsters, cushions, or blocks. Inhale and take both arms overhead onto the floor behind you. Exhale and return the arms back to the starting position. You can silently coordinate the breath and movement with the affirmation. Inhale and affirm, *Love blossoms.* Exhale and affirm, *With each breath.* Repeat 6 times.

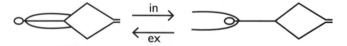

Supine Butterfly Pose with arm movements

14. *Pelvic Flower Exercise in Supine Butterfly Pose* (Supta Baddha Konasana)

It's important to keep the pelvic floor strong, but at the same time it's also important to know how to relax it. This exercise will help you relax the pelvic floor and can also enhance sexual enjoyment. Lie on your back in Supine Butterfly Pose (*Supta Baddha Konasana*). Rest your hands either on your belly or above your head. Imagine that there is a beautiful flower between your legs, at the pelvic floor: as you inhale the flower opens and as you exhale the flower closes back to bud. Repeat for a few breaths. Be present to any sensations that arise in the pelvic floor area as you do this exercise.

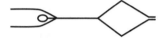

Pelvic Flower Exercise in Supine Butterfly Pose

15. *Full-Body Stretch*

From Supine Butterfly Pose (*Supta Baddha Konasana*), stretch both legs out along the floor and take both arms overhead. Lengthen tall along the floor. Stay for a few breaths.

Either finish your practice here or move on to step 16.

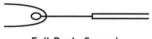

Full-Body Stretch

16. *Universal Wind-Down Routine*

Perform the Universal Wind-Down Routine from chapter 1.

17. *Om Mani Padme Hum, plus Lotus Flower Visualization*

If you have time, do the Om Mani Padme Hum, Plus Lotus Flower Visualization on page 86. It is a wonderful way to conclude this yoga practice. You can also use your own favorite relaxation or meditation.

Taurus-Inspired Yoga Practice Overview

1. Easy Pose hands in Prayer Position. Blossom visualization, with affirmation: *Love blossoms with each breath.*

2. Cat Pose into Cow Pose × 8.

3. Wave to the Moon Pose × 6. Repeat on other side.

4. Heart Chakra Sequence with mantra *Yam* × 6.

5. Lunge Pose with arm movements × 4. On final movement, stay in open-chest position for a few breaths. Repeat other side.

6. Downward-Facing Dog Pose into a Standing Forward Bend. Stay for a few breaths in both poses. Uncurl and come back up to standing.

7. Standing like a tree in blossom. Stay for a few breaths, repeating affirmation: *Love blossoms with each breath.*

8. Tree Pose. Stay for a few breaths. Repeat on other side.

9. Blossom Petal Sequence.

10. Lunge Pose with Twist × 4. Repeat on other side.

11. Child's Pose into Upward-Facing Dog × 6. Coordinate breath and movement with affirmation. Inhale: *Love blossoms.* Exhale: *With each breath.*

12. Seated Forward Bend. Coordinate breath and movement with affirmation. Inhale: *Love blossoms.* Exhale: *With each breath.* Repeat × 6, on final time stay a few breaths in pose.

13. Supine Butterfly Pose with arm movements. Coordinate breath and movement with affirmation. Inhale: *Love blossoms.* Exhale: *With each breath.* Repeat × 6.

14. Pelvic Flower Exercise in Supine Butterfly Pose with flower visualization.

15. Full-Body Stretch. Stay for a few breaths. *Finish here or move on to step 16.*

16. Universal Wind-Down Routine.

17. *Om Mani Padme Hum,* Plus Lotus Flower Visualization or your own relaxation.

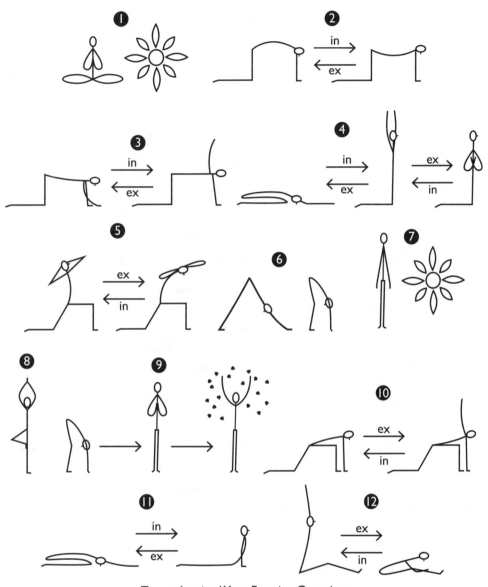

Taurus-Inspired Yoga Practice Overview

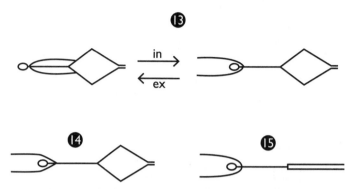

Taurus-Inspired Yoga Practice Overview (continued)

<hr>

VISUALIZATION

Om Mani Padme Hum, Plus Lotus Flower

This meditation has been chosen because it fits in with the themes of beauty, love, harmony, and blossoming, which are associated with Venus, the ruling planet of Taurus.

Om mani padme hum is the central phrase of Tantrism and can be translated as "the jewel in the lotus." In Asia the lotus is often personified as the goddess Padma.[26] The lotus (*padma*) is the symbol of spiritual unfoldment or blossoming.[27]

If you are not familiar with the chant, you can check it out online. I particularly like Jane Winther's rendering of *Om mani padme hum*, which can be found on YouTube.

When we combine the mantra with the lotus flower visualization, it promotes a sense of open-heartedness and compassion.

The meditation begins with picturing a lotus fully open, which helps us cultivate a sense of blossoming on a physical, emotional, and spiritual level. We conclude the meditation by picturing the flower closing back to bud, which creates a sense of psychic protection and safety. Whereas in meditation it can be very

<hr>

26. Walker, *The Woman's Encyclopedia of Myths and Secrets*, 549–50.

27. Georg Feuerstein, *The Yoga Tradition: Its History, Literature, Philosophy and Practice* (Prescott, AZ: Holm Press, 2001), 177.

therapeutic and uplifting to fully open and blossom, in everyday life we some-times need to be able to put on an extra layer of psychic protection. In this way the image of a flower closing back to bud is a good way to conclude a yoga or meditation practice, as it helps with the transition back to a safe level of openness for resuming everyday life.

This meditation can be done sitting down or lying down. Allow 5 to 10 minutes.

To start off, bring your awareness to your heart center and maintain a gentle, background awareness of your heart center throughout the meditation.

Begin to silently repeat the mantra *Om mani padme hum*. Repeat several times, until you feel your body, mind, and feelings begin to settle.

Now picture a lotus flower floating on a calm, still pool. The flower is bathed in sunlight, its petals are open, and a droplet of dew glows jewellike, cupped inside the flower.

Hold this image of the lotus flower in your mind's eye for a few more breaths, and at the same time maintain a gentle background awareness of your heart cen-ter and the natural flow of your breath.

When you feel ready, picture the flower closing back to bud, and then let go of the image of the flower.

Repeat the mantra *Om mani padme hum* a few more times, either chanting it out loud or repeating it silently to yourself.

Let go of chanting the mantra and come back to simply observing the natu-ral flow of the breath. Then let go of following the breath and notice where your body is in contact with the floor, or your support, and the sensations associated with this.

Take some time to notice what effect doing this meditation has had upon you. Resolve to take this sense of spiritual blossoming into whatever you do today.

Taurus-Inspired Meditation Questions

See chapter 1 for guidance on how to use meditation questions. The theme is "blossom-ing to your full potential."

- What is beautiful in my life and brings me joy?
- How do I create the right conditions for love to blossom in my life?
- How do I nurture my creativity?

- Do I have any hidden talents that I would like to develop and grow?
- What are the obstacles standing in the way of reaching my full potential in life?
    - What steps could I take to overcome these obstacles?
- Which yoga poses help me release, relax, open, unfold, and blossom?
- Which meditative practices help increase my clarity and allow my awareness to blossom?
- How do I help others find joy in their life and help them blossom too?

CHAPTER 6

Yoga Takes You Higher

♊
Gemini

May 20–June 21
Unite your Sun and Moon energies,
ignite your spark of genius, and let your spirit soar!

Sunlight and shadow are integral aspects of our yoga practice. Yoga philosophy tells us that we can find the Sun, the Moon, the planets, and all the stars within our own body. The Sun is in the belly, and the Moon above the crown of the head. *Prana* manifests within the subtle body as both Sun and Moon energies. The spine is the Tree of Life with the Sun on one side, and the Moon on the other. Our yoga practice brings these two energies together, and heaven and earth are reunited.

Within each of us there is a spark of genius. Through yoga we access this divine inspiration and let it fly high and wide. Yogis believe that the air we breathe contains *prana*. It is the subtle energy that powers all of creation, including you, me, the Sun, the Moon, and the stars. *Prana* is life force, spirit, and intelligence combined. The breath is the key to inspiration, to unlocking the spirit and letting it take flight.

Spirit, mind, intelligence, vitality, and energy are all intertwined with the breath. By connecting with the breath, we are connecting to life itself. *Pranayama* is sometimes translated to "breath control"; however, trying to control the breath is about as possible as attempting to control the wind or turn back the waves. Our yoga breathing practices teach us to ride, respect, and listen to the breath. We learn to observe, follow, and be guided by it. In turn we are carried higher on the wings of the breath.

Our yoga practice is powered by air, powered by *prana*. We learn to follow the lead of the breath. Each movement we make is surrounded by breath and infused with *prana*. On the inhalation, the lungs fill with air like balloons. We are energized and revitalized. On the exhalation, we let go of impurities. Our system is cleansed, blockages are removed, and vital energy can be transported around our body without any impediment. Breath is linked to body, to mind, to emotions, and to spirit. The breath is the teacher and the guru.

When you conjure up an image of a yogi, perhaps you think of an ascetic alone in a cave in the Himalayas meditating for years at a time. This is one aspect of yoga, but yoga is also about relationship. It helps us connect and communicate with others.

Sometimes it is good to be silent and quieten down the noise—to come offline, to disconnect from the virtual world of cyberspace, and to reconnect with the space within your own heart. At other times it's good to get your ideas out into the world, to speak out, to share your life and your opinions, and to inspire others. Yoga gives you the clarity to get your point of view across. Nowadays, thanks to modern technology, there are so many ways that our ideas, like seed heads, can be carried on the wind and communicated to others.

Yoga teaches us to reconcile differences, to appreciate both sunlight and shadow. We choose to focus on what connects us to others, not on what separates us. By uniting the energies of heaven and earth, Sun and Moon, energy is freed, our spirit soars, and our wings open.

Yoga Inspired by Gemini

The Egyptian symbol of Gemini was a woman and man holding hands. In Sanskrit, they were called *Maithuna*, the Lovers.[28] The symbol of the twins resonates with a central tenet of yoga philosophy, which is the idea of uniting complementary opposites, such as Sun and Moon, masculine and feminine, night and day, dark and light, action and rest,

---

28. Walker, *The Woman's Dictionary of Symbols and Sacred Objects*, 290.

stillness and movement, earth and heaven. In the Gemini-inspired yoga practice that follows we explore duality by integrating Sun and Moon imagery into our practice.

Gemini is ruled by the planet Mercury, and its key word is *communication*. Mercury governs arts, sciences, and all kinds of knowledge. It is the ruling planet of the internet, mobile phones, television, radio, and other means of communication. Retrograde Mercury is when the planet Mercury at certain times of the year appears to be going backward. Some people blame this occurrence for glitches in technology, such as their phone, laptop, or other gadgets malfunctioning. However, although it's fun to look upon the planet Mercury as some sort of planetary gremlin that hexes our technological devices, there is no science in it, as Mercury does not actually change direction: it's just an optical illusion.[29]

Mercury was the swift messenger of the gods. Air is the element associated with Gemini, which fits in perfectly with the imagery of the winged feet and helmet that we use in the yoga practice that follows. It's fun and exhilarating to perform yoga poses while imagining that you have wings. The winged power of Mercury lifts you higher; you overcome obstacles and feel that anything is possible. You find yourself achieving poses that were previously beyond your grasp.

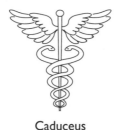

Caduceus

In Greece Mercury was known as Hermes. He carried the caduceus, a magic wand that could control the elements and transform whatever it touched into gold. This ancient symbol is known in many cultures and is associated with magical and healing powers. It is still an international symbol for both the medical profession and homeopaths.

You would be forgiven for thinking that contemplation upon the symbolism of a Greek god's magic wand has taken us a long way from yoga. However, we come full circle back to our yoga roots with the realization that in Hindu symbolism the caduceus is

---

29. Karen Zraick, "Mercury Is in Retrograde. Don't Be Alarmed," *New York Times*, March 14, 2019, https://www.nytimes.com/2019/03/14/style/mercury-retrograde-facts.html.

equated with the central spirit of the human body, the spinal column with the two mystic serpents twined around it, *ida-nadi* to the left and *pingala-nadi* to the right.[30] The esoteric anatomy of the ancient yogis centered around three primary channels (*nadis*), which were conduits of the life force (*prana*). The central channel, the *sushumna,* ran through the center of the spine, and on either side were to be found the cooling Moon channel (*ida-nadi*) and the heating Sun channel (*pingala-nadi*). To achieve self-realization, the serpent energy (*kundalini*), had to ascend from the base chakra, through the sushumna, to the chakra at the crown of the head.[31]

I knew all the above, but it had always seemed just an academic concept to me. However, meditating upon the symbol of the caduceus in preparation for creating a Gemini-inspired yoga practice changed all that for me. A veil was lifted, and I could perceive the subtle energy channels, carrying the life force as a real, tangible, and beautiful reality. I found that a good way to meditate on the symbol of the caduceus was to picture a tree of life, with the Sun and Moon on either side, and to picture myself as that tree, with my spine at the center, and flanked by the Sun and Moon. From here the wings, to be found at the tip of the caduceus wand, easily transform into higher consciousness, the state of bliss, self-realization, *samadhi.*

We also develop further the Gemini theme of uniting complementary opposites in the Sun and Moon Meditation that follows later in this chapter.

Gemini-Inspired Yoga Practice

The Gemini-inspired yoga practice that follows is suitable for everyone, regardless of their sign. It's energizing, elevating, and uplifting. It will help you transcend your sense of limitation, overcome difficulties, and open to new possibilities. It balances and harmonizes our Sun and Moon energies and creates a sense of peaceful elation.

The affirmation we use in the practice is *All is possible with wisdom and compassion.* It can be shortened and coordinated with the breath:

Inhale: Wisdom

Exhale: Compassion

Allow 25 to 35 minutes.

---

30. Walker, *The Woman's Encyclopedia of Myths and Secrets,* 131.

31. Feuerstein, *Encyclopedic Dictionary of Yoga,* 143, 228, 259, and 354.

1. Sun and moon visualization seated

Find yourself a comfortable seated position. Sit tall and drop your awareness down to your belly, picturing a warm sun there radiating love and compassion. Then take your awareness to the space just above the crown of your head. Picture a cool, clear moon there, and imagine the moon's clarity filling you with penetrating wisdom. Keep coming back to this sun and moon imagery throughout the practice.

Silently repeat this affirmation: *All is possible with wisdom and compassion.*

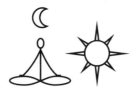

Sun and moon visualization

2. Cat Pose (Marjaryasana) *into Cow Pose* (Bitilasana)

Start on all fours. Exhaling, round the back up like an angry cat. Inhale into Cow Pose (*Bitilasana*), arching the back, lifting the chest up and away from the belly, and look-ing up slightly. Alternate between these two positions, rounding and arching the back. Repeat 8 times. (If you have a back problem, don't arch the back).

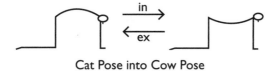

Cat Pose into Cow Pose

3. Flying Cat Pose (Marjaryasana *variation*)

Start on all fours. Imagine that your feet have wings. Exhaling, round the back up, bring-ing one knee toward the head. Inhaling, straighten the leg out behind you and keep the pelvis level. Repeat 6 times on this side, visualizing that the feet are winged. Repeat on the other side.

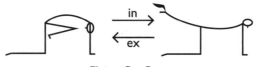

Flying Cat Pose

4. *Mountain Pose* (Tadasana) *with sun and moon visualization*

Stand tall, feet parallel and about hip width apart. Next drop your awareness down to your belly. Picture a warm sun there, radiating love and compassion. Then take your awareness to the space just above the crown of your head. Picture a cool, clear moon there, and imagine the moon's clarity filling you with penetrating wisdom.

Silently repeat this affirmation: *All is possible with wisdom and compassion.*

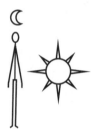

Mountain Pose with sun and moon visualization

5. *Dancer Pose with winged feet* (Natarajasana *variation*)

Stand tall, feet hip width apart, arms by your sides. Imagine that both your feet have wings (and if you wish, you could imagine you have a winged helmet too). Bend your right knee, and with your right hand catch hold of your ankle. Take the left arm up above the head. From here, tip the torso forward, extend your winged back foot away from you, and reach forward and up with the opposite arm. Stay for a few breaths. Repeat on the other side. If you have balance problems, practice facing a wall, with your extended hand resting on the wall for support.

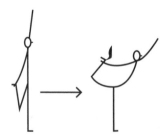

Dancer Pose with winged feet

6. *Intense Side Stretch Pose with winged feet* (Parsvottanasana *variation*)

Stand tall, feet hip width apart. Imagine that both your feet have wings (and if you wish, you could imagine you have a winged helmet too). Step one foot forward. Inhaling, take the arms up above the head and slightly bend the front knee. Exhaling, bend forward over the front leg, lowering your fingertips to the floor. Inhaling, lift your back winged foot from the floor, raising the leg to hip height or higher. Exhaling, lower the foot back to the floor. Then as you inhale, come back up, raising the arms above the head. Repeat 3 times, and then repeat on the other side.

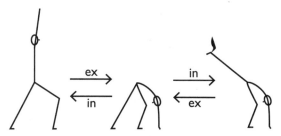

Intense Side Stretch Pose with winged feet

7. *Flying Dog Pose* (**Adho Mukha Svanasana** *variation*)

On your final time in Intense Side Stretch Pose (*Parsvottanasana*), place both hands on the floor, on either side of the front foot, and step back into Downward-Facing Dog Pose (*Adho Mukha Svanasana*). Establish yourself comfortably in Downward-Facing Dog Pose, maintaining the imagery of winged feet, and then lift one straight leg to hip height; if that feels okay, lift the leg higher so that it is in line with the torso. Do not tilt the pelvis. Repeat on the other side. Repeat 4 times on each side.

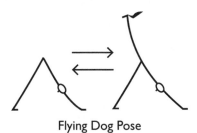

Flying Dog Pose

8. *Boat Pose with winged feet* (**Navasana** *variation*)

Sit with your legs outstretched in front of you, knees bent and heels resting on the floor. Imagine that both your feet have wings (and if you wish, picture a winged helmet too). Lean backward slightly, keeping a long back, with your head and neck in line with the spine and your lower abs gently pulling back toward the spine. Lift the winged heels from the floor and raise the legs to make a V shape out of your body. For an easier pose keep the legs slightly bent. Don't round the back. As you hold the pose, silently repeat this affirmation: *All is possible with wisdom and compassion.*

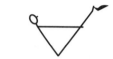

Boat Pose with winged feet

9. *Bow Pose variation* (**Dhanurasana** *variation*)

Lie on your front with your arms by your sides. Inhaling, lift your chest as you bend both knees. Exhaling, lower the chest and straighten your legs back to the floor. Repeat 6 times, staying in the final pose for a few breaths.

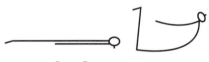

Bow Pose variation

If you wish to work at a gentler level, skip step 10 and go straight to Child's Pose, or repeat Bow Pose variation once more.

10. *Bow Pose with winged feet* (**Dhanurasana**)

Lie on your front with your arms by your sides. Imagine that both your feet have wings (and if you wish, you could imagine you have a winged helmet too). Bend both knees and catch hold of your ankles. Lift your chest and knees up and away from the floor, gently pulling your shoulders back to open the chest. If comfortable, stay here for a few breaths. Then lower down to the floor, release the ankles, straighten your legs along the floor, and turn your head to one side, resting for a few breaths.

Bow Pose with winged feet

11. *Cat Pose* (Marjaryasana) *into Child's Pose* (Balasana)

Come onto all fours. Exhaling, lower the bottom to the heels and the head to the floor into Child's Pose (*Balasana*). Inhaling, come back up to all fours. Repeat 6 times. As you inhale, silently say, *Wisdom*, and on the exhale, *Compassion*.

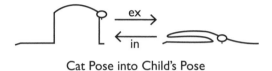

Cat Pose into Child's Pose

12. *Child's Pose* (Balasana)

Rest for a few breaths here.

Child's Pose

13. *Lying on the back, with knees bent and feet on floor*

Close your eyes and let go of the imagery of winged feet and a winged helmet. Imagine that where the wings have been attached there are flowers, and visualize each flower closing back to bud.

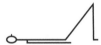

Lying on the back, with knees bent and feet on floor

14. *Supine Butterfly Pose with arm movements* (**Supta Baddha Konasana** *variation*)

Lie on your back, knees spread out to the sides and soles of feet together, with your hands resting on your belly or tops of the thighs. For comfort prop your knees on bolsters, cushions, or blocks. Inhale: take both arms overhead onto the floor behind you. Exhaling, return the arms back to the starting position. You can silently coordinate the breath and movement with the affirmation. Inhale and affirm, *All is possible.* Exhale and affirm, *With wisdom and compassion.* Repeat 6 times.

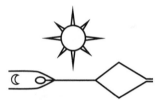

Supine Butterfly Pose with arm movements

15. *Supine Butterfly Pose* (**Supta Baddha Konasana**), *with sun and moon visualization*

Drop your awareness down to your belly. Picture a warm sun there, radiating love and compassion. Then take your awareness to the space just above the crown of your head. Picture a cool, clear moon there, and imagine the moon's clarity filling you with penetrating wisdom. Silently repeat this affirmation: *All is possible with wisdom and compassion.*

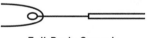

Supine Butterfly Pose with sun and moon visualization

16. *Full-Body Stretch*

Lengthen tall along the floor. Stay for a few breaths. *If you are short of time, finish here or do the Universal Wind-Down Routine in chapter 1.*

Full-Body Stretch

17. *Short relaxation or Sun and Moon Meditation*

Either finish with a short relaxation or, if you have more time, do the Sun and Moon Meditation on page 101.

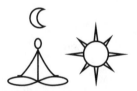

Sun and Moon Meditation

Gemini-Inspired Yoga Practice Overview

1. Sun and moon visualization with affirmation: *All is possible with wisdom and compassion.*

2. Cat Pose into Cow Pose × 8.

3. Flying Cat Pose × 6. Repeat on other side.

4. Mountain Pose with sun and moon visualization and affirmation: *All is possible with wisdom and compassion.*

5. Dancer Pose with winged feet. Stay a few breaths and repeat on other side.

6. Intense Side Stretch Pose with winged feet. Repeat × 3, and then repeat on other side.

7. Flying Dog Pose. Leg lifts on each side × 4.

8. Boat Pose with winged feet. Hold the pose, silently repeating affirmation: *All is possible with wisdom and compassion.*

9. Bow Pose variation. Repeat × 6. Stay in the final pose for a few breaths.

10. Bow Pose with winged feet. If comfortable, stay here for a few breaths.

11. Cat Pose into Child's Pose. Repeat 6 times. Inhale: *Wisdom.* Exhale: *Compassion.*

12. Child's Pose (*Balasana*). Rest for a few breaths here.

13. Lie on back, knees bent, feet on floor. Flower closing back to bud visualization.

14. Supine Butterfly Pose with arm movements. Inhale: *All is possible.* Exhale: *With wisdom and compassion.* Repeat × 6.

15. Supine Butterfly Pose and sun and moon visualization with affirmation: *All is possible with wisdom and compassion.*

16. Full-Body Stretch: stay for a few breaths. *If you are short of time, finish here or do the Universal Wind-Down Routine.*

17. Short relaxation or Sun and Moon Meditation.

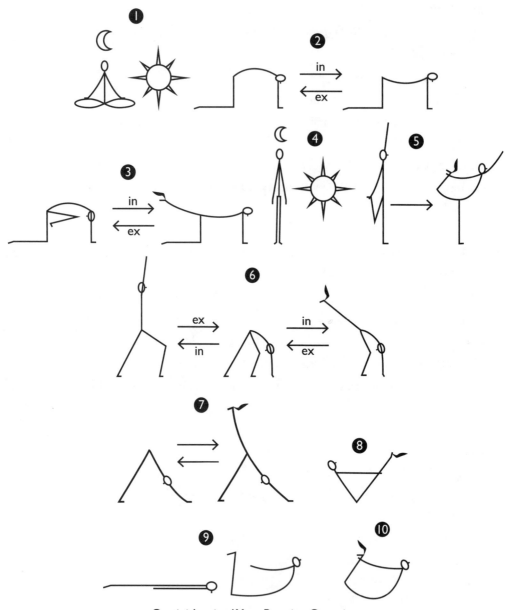

Gemini-Inspired Yoga Practice Overview

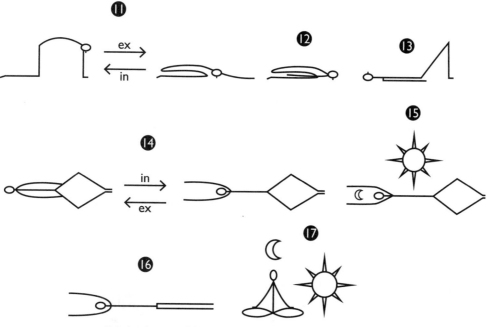

Gemini-Inspired Yoga Practice Overview (continued)

MEDITATION

Sun and Moon

This meditation has been chosen because its use of sun and moon imagery fits in with the Gemini theme of uniting complementary opposites.

The meditation is divided into two parts. The first part, Getting into Your Pole, can be used anytime that you want to ground, center, and align yourself. I first learned this technique in the context of a women's self-defense course. It creates a sense of steadiness and empowerment. It can be used anytime, on or off the mat, sitting or standing. It will help you get back on track when you've been emotionally thrown off balance. It's also useful in situations when you need to assert yourself. I use it at the start of my home yoga practice, standing in Mountain Pose (*Tadasana*), and before I commence teaching a yoga class.

The second part of the meditation, Uniting Sun and Moon Energies, will help you connect with and unite your subtle sun and moon energies, which creates the right conditions for a blissful sense of being at one with it all to arise.

Step One: Getting into Your Pole

Find yourself a comfortable, erect sitting position, either on the floor or sitting on an upright chair.

Notice where your body is in contact with the floor or your support. Allow yourself to relax into this support, while at the same time feeling yourself growing tall.

Become aware of your spine; feel into the spine, taking your awareness from the base of the spine up to the crown of your head. Now imagine that there is a pole that runs through the center of your spine connecting you to the earth below and to the sky above. Picture this pole descending from your tailbone, traveling down deep into the earth, and simultaneously ascending high up into the sky above from the crown of your head. Feel that you are connected to the earth below and to heaven above.

Step Two: Uniting Sun and Moon Energies

Drop your awareness down to your belly. Picture a warm sun there, radiating love and compassion. Then take your awareness to the space just above the crown of your head. Picture a cool, clear moon there, and imagine the moon's clarity filling you with penetrating wisdom.

Bring your awareness back to your spine and picture the spinal column as a channel that unites the sun energy at your belly and the moon energy at the crown of your head. Imagine the energetic connection running along the length of your spine, uniting the fiery, compassionate sun energy and the cool, penetrating wisdom of the moon energy. Allow yourself to relax into the blissful union of these two energies.

Now let go of the image of the sun and the moon. Where you were picturing the moon above the head, imagine a fully open lotus flower. Picture this flower closing back to bud. And where you were picturing the sun at the belly, imagine a red, yellow, or orange flower fully open, and then picture it closing back to bud. Then let go of the image of the flowers.

Once again, become aware of your spine; notice how the spine gently undulates with each in- and out-breath. Allow your spine to be moved by the breath. Particularly, be aware of the base of the skull and the tailbone moving toward and away from each other with each inhalation and exhalation.

To conclude the meditation simply notice where your body is in contact with the floor or your support, and notice any sensations associated with this. Become aware of the sounds inside and outside the room and be fully present to your body sitting here and your immediate surroundings.

Spend a few moments considering any insights that have arisen for you during this meditation, and if you want to, write them down.

Gemini-Inspired Meditation Questions

See chapter 1 for guidance on how to use the meditation questions. The theme is "connecting with your genius and shining your light out into the world."

- What do I find uplifting and energizing in my life?
- When I am feeling heavy and low, which yoga poses lift my mood and take me higher?
  - Which meditation practices do the same?
- Are there any pairs of opposites in my life that need reconciling and healing?
- How do I best create balance in my life between my active Sun energy and my relaxing Moon energy?
  - Which yoga practices would help me achieve this balance?
- How does my own unique spark of genius manifest? (Forget about being modest for the moment!)
  - What gets in the way of me shining my light out into the world?
  - How do I overcome this?
- What are my favorite ways of communicating my ideas to others?
  - How could I improve my communication skills and make them more effective?
- How do I help others uncover their own unique genius and shine it out into the world?

CHAPTER 7

Creating Your Sanctuary

Cancer

June 21–July 22

Nurture and nourish yourself away from the fray of life and take time out for healing.

The path of yoga is a path that will lead you home to yourself. When the world feels hostile and unwelcoming, yoga is a place of sanctuary. When you feel unwanted, unloved, or uncared for, it provides a place of refuge. Step onto your yoga mat and you are stepping into sacred space. Here you are loved; you can let the public mask slip and simply be yourself.

Yoga breathes you. She is the umbilical cord connecting you to the source of life. She gives you the milk of human kindness. Like a mother concerned for her only child, she will attend to whatever arises for you. If your body is tired, heavy, aching, or in pain, she will find the yoga pose that is the balm to heal you. If you are troubled or your feelings are hurt, she will find the words to comfort and soothe you. She will smooth the worry lines from your brow, relax your shoulders down away from your ears, unclench your fist, and give you rest.

You are held in the circle of yoga. The circle is strong enough to hold whatever burdens you are carrying. Yoga teaches us to relax into the support that life can offer. We are held, nurtured, and nourished. The water on the surface of your life might be turbulent, but underneath the pool is deep, calm, and still.

When life bites you, yoga will reveal to you the wisdom and learning that lies within the wound and show you the medicine that is needed to heal. She gives you a space to find healing away from the fray of life. When your heart is contracted and closed, refusing to let life in, she coaxes you to take a breath in and a breath out. Each in-breath, each out-breath connects you to the pulse of life, and once again you are back in the flow of life, the flow of love.

Do not push away worry or "negative" feelings; rather, attend to these feelings as you would a crying baby that needs comforting. Look after the fretful child within and soothe her with comforting words and a warm, loving attitude.

Whenever you feel anxious or not at home, feel the earth beneath your feet giving you support. When worry energy makes you feel ill at ease and disconnected, the Mountain Pose (*Tadasana*) will help you feel your connection to Mother Earth. In the pose bring your awareness down to your feet, feel roots from the feet connecting you to the earth, grounding your energy, and helping you feel supported.

In each asana be aware of where your body is in contact with the earth. Breathe out and relax into the support of the earth beneath you; breathe in and feel yourself energized by the earth. This will help you come home to yourself.

With time and experience we become more adept at choosing the right asana to bring healing. When we feel frazzled and overstimulated, we take time out in Child's Pose (*Balasana*) or relax into a Seated Forward Bend (*Paschimottanasana*). When an unhappy experience has made us close off from life, a backward bend such as Cobra Pose (*Bhujangasana*) will open our heart up to the enjoyment of life again. When we feel stuck and unable to move forward, the energy of water helps us flow in and out of our yoga poses, and soon our life is flowing again. We learn the gentle discipline of simply being.

In each yoga posture, we are carried, nurtured, and nourished by the breath. We learn to ride the waves of the breath, and in this way, we feel supported. There is nowhere to get to, nothing to do, no need to become anything other than what we already are. We are a heart beating, a body breathing, held in blue-sky consciousness—spacious, open, and entirely at home.

Yoga Inspired by the Zodiac Sign Cancer

Cancer, the crab, is a water sign ruled by the Moon. It is known as the mother sign, with a strong desire to care for, nourish, and protect others. The parts of the body associated with it are the breasts, the stomach, and the digestive system (all to do with feeding and nourishment). It is a homely sign, associated with anything enclosed that surrounds and protects, including the womb, the cradle, and the grave. The private and the hidden are concerns for this sign. Key words are *sensitively* and *protectively*.

Our spiritual practice trains us to embrace the parts of ourselves that we would rather keep private and hidden. Cancer, the sign of the crab, gives us the opportunity to scrutinize where in our life we are showing crab-like tendencies by erecting a hard shell of defensiveness to protect our soft, vulnerable heart. The mother imagery of the sign enables us to use our nurturing skills (available to all genders), to develop the courage and compassion to accept ourselves as we are, in the here and now. So although the strong, sharp pinch from a crab's claw may seem a "negative" image, it can be a reminder for us to let go of our ideals and embrace our lives as they are now, with all their imperfection and exquisite beauty. When that happens, we will truly come home to ourselves.

This sign gives us the opportunity to look at the nurturing, nourishing side of motherly love, while simultaneously the sharp pinch of the crab's claw reminds us not to fall into the trap of reducing motherhood to a sentimental ideal. The Indian goddess Kali Ma mirrors this dual aspect of mother as both creator and destroyer. Similarly, Mother Earth is the ground we walk upon; she supports us, provides us with food and shelter, and gives us water when we are thirsty and rest when we are tired. She is a gentle, kind, loving mother and at the same time, she is also a fierce mother who can kill us with earthquakes, tornadoes, hurricanes, and erupting volcanoes. Like the goddess Kali Ma, she is to be loved, respected, and feared!

Kali Ma also sometimes manifests as Durga, a warrior queen who personifies the fighting spirit of a mother protecting her young. As the goddess of both creation and destruction, Kali Ma provides a good metaphor for the complexity of feelings that we have, both as a society and as individuals, toward our mothers and the concept of motherhood.

In the practice that follows we use the mantra *Ma* to induce a sense of well-being and connectedness. *Ma* is the basic mother syllable of Indo-European languages. In the Far East it represents the "spark of life" and was often defined as intelligence.[32] We use the

---

32. Walker, *The Woman's Encyclopedia of Myths and Secrets*, 560.

seed mantra *Vam*, which is associated with the second chakra (*svadhisthana*), to reflect the watery nature of this sign, ruled by the Moon.

We also integrate into the practice the yogic concept of withdrawal of the senses (*pratyahara*) to enable us to access a place within us that is an island, a refuge from the storm. Poses such as Tortoise Pose (*Kurmasana*), allow us to draw our awareness inward, to take time out, and to just simply be in our own private, peaceful haven. It's a wonderful antidote to lives that are lived out in the public glare of social media. Pure bliss!

The practice concludes with the Become Your Own Best Friend Meditation, chosen because it relates to the Cancer sign's themes of motherly love and learning to nurture and nourish ourselves.

Cancer-Inspired Yoga Practice

The Cancer-inspired practice that follows aims to create a nourishing, nurturing space that will help you to feel at home and comfortable in your own skin. When you arrive in the present moment, you will feel a sense of coming home to yourself.

The affirmation we use in the practice is *I am home in the here and now.*

It can be shortened and coordinated with the breath:

Inhale: I am home

Exhale: Here and now

Allow 20 to 30 minutes.

1. *Mountain Pose* (Tadasana)

Stand tall, feet parallel and about hip width apart. Be aware of the contact between your feet and the earth beneath you. Imagine a string attached to the crown of your head, gently pulling you skyward; simultaneously, let your tailbone drop and feel your heels rooting down into the earth. Silently repeat this affirmation: *I am home in the here and now.*

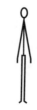

Mountain Pose

2. *Flower arms*

Stand tall, feet hip width apart. Place your fingertips on your shoulders, elbows out to the sides; relax your shoulders down away from ears. Inhaling, open the arms out to the sides like a flower opening. Exhaling, bend the arms, bringing the fingertips back to the shoulders like a flower closing back to bud. You can coordinate the breath with the affirmation. Inhale and affirm, *I am home.* Exhale and affirm, *Here and now.* Repeat 6 times.

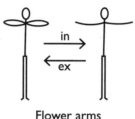

Flower arms

3. *Albatross Sequence 1*

Stand tall, feet hip width apart. Inhaling, raise the arms above the head. Exhaling, bend forward about 45 degrees with your back slightly arched and arms spread out to the sides like a bird's wings (this is Albatross Pose). Stay for one breath in the pose. Inhaling, come back up to standing, sweeping the arms above the head. Exhaling, lower the arms back to the sides. Repeat the sequence 4 to 6 times.

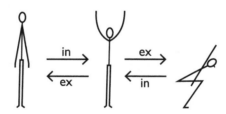

Albatross Sequence 1

4. *Warrior 1* (Virabhadrasana 1) *variation*

Stand tall, feet hip width apart, turn your left foot slightly out, and take a big step forward with your right leg. Place your hands on your belly, feeling a sense of coming home to yourself. Inhaling, bend your right knee, opening your arms out wide to the side. Exhaling, straighten your right leg and bring your hands back to your belly. You can coordinate the breath with the affirmation. Inhale and affirm, *I am home.* Exhale and affirm, *Here and now.* Do 6 repetitions on this side and then repeat on the other side.

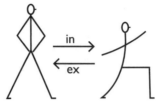

Warrior I variation

5. *Warrior 1* (Virabhadrasana 1)

Stand tall, feet hip width apart, turn your left foot slightly out, and take a big step forward with your right leg. Take both arms overhead, bringing the palms of the hands together (for a gentler pose have the hands shoulder width apart). Silently repeat this affirmation 3 times: *I am home in the here and now.*

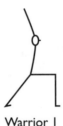

Warrior I

6. *Albatross Sequence 2*

Stand tall, feet hip width apart and hands resting on your belly. Inhaling, raise the arms. Exhaling, sweep the arms out to the sides like a bird's wings as you bend halfway forward, back slightly arched, into Albatross Pose. Stay here and inhale. Exhaling, lower into Standing Forward Bend (*Uttanasana*). Inhaling, bend the knees and arch the back. Exhale back down into a forward bend. Inhaling, sweep arms out to the side and up above the head as you come back up to standing. Exhaling, lower the hands back to belly. Repeat the sequence 4 times.

Albatross Sequence 2

7. *Mantra* Ma *Sequence 1*

Come to tall kneeling, hands in the Prayer Position (*Namaste*). Inhale and raise the arms. Exhale and sound the mantra *Ma* as you fold forward into Child's Pose (*Balasana*), arms outstretched along the floor. Inhaling, come back to tall kneeling with arms raised. Exhaling, bring hands back into prayer position. Repeat the sequence 4 to 6 times.

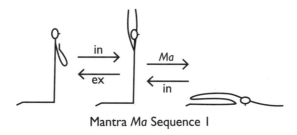

Mantra *Ma* Sequence I

8a. *Supine Twist* (Jathara Parivrtti)

Lie on your back, knees bent, feet together, arms out to the sides at shoulder height, and palms facing down. Bring both knees onto your chest (for an easier pose keep both feet on the floor). Exhaling, lower both knees down toward the floor on the left; turn your head gently to the right. Inhale and return to center. With each exhale, silently repeat the mantra *Vam* (pronounced *vum*). Allow your movements to be flowing and watery. Repeat 6 times on each side, alternating sides.

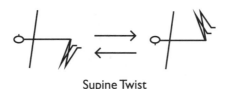

Supine Twist

8b. *Supine Twist* (Jathara Parivrtti) *continued*

Drop your knees to the left and place your left hand atop your right thigh, gently persuading your legs nearer to the floor. Turn your right palm up and, keeping your arm in contact with the floor, raise your arm up toward your right ear. At the end of each exhale silently repeat the mantra *Vam* (pronounced *vum*). Stay here for a few breaths, and then repeat on the other side.

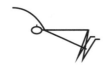

Supine Twist continued

9. *Seated Forward Bend* (Paschimottanasana)

Sit tall, legs outstretched (bend the knees to ease the pose). Inhaling, raise the arms. Exhale and fold forward over the legs. Inhale and return to starting position. You can silently coordinate the breath and movement with the affirmation. Inhale and affirm, *I am home.* Exhale and affirm, *Here and now.* Repeat 6 times, and on the final time stay for a few breaths in the pose.

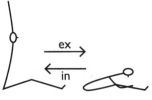

Seated Forward Bend

10. *Tortoise Pose* (Kurmasana)

Sit tall, legs just over hip width apart and knees bent. Lower the torso into a forward bend. Slip both arms under the knees and behind you to rest on the lower back. For an easier alternative, catch hold of the outside of the ankles. Stay for a few breaths, drawing your awareness inward. To work more gently, skip this pose or do a Seated Forward Bend (*Paschimottanasana*) instead.

Tortoise Pose

11. *Mantra* Ma *Sequence 2*

Come to tall kneeling, hands in the Prayer Position (Namaste). Inhale and raise the arms. Exhale and sound the mantra *Ma* as you fold forward into Child's Pose (*Balasana*), arms outstretched along the floor. From Child's Pose inhale and move forward into Upward-Facing Dog (*Urdhva Mukha Svanasana*), arching your back and keeping your knees on the floor. Exhale back into Child's Pose. Inhaling, come back to tall kneeling with arms raised. Exhale and bring hands into Prayer Position. Repeat the sequence 4 to 6 times.

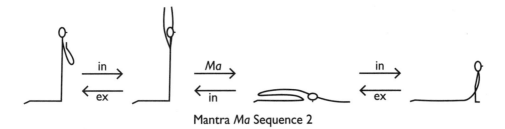

Mantra *Ma* Sequence 2

12. *Bridge Pose* (Setu Bandhasana) *with arm movements*

Lie on your back with your knees bent and feet hip width apart. Inhaling, slowly peel the back from the floor and raise the arms above the head. Exhaling, lower the back to the floor and simultaneously lower the arms. Inhale and affirm, *I am home.* Exhale and affirm, *Here and now.* Repeat 6 times, staying for a few breaths the final time.

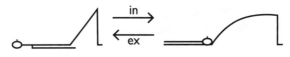

Bridge Pose with arm movements

13. *Knees-to-Chest Pose* (Apanasana)

Hug the knees into the chest. Rest here for a few breaths. Silently repeat 3 times the affirmation: *I am home in the here and now.*

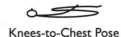

Knees-to-Chest Pose

14. *Full-Body Stretch*

Lying on your back, stretch both legs out along the floor and take both arms overhead. Lengthen tall along the floor. Stay for a few breaths.

If you are short of time, finish here with a few minutes of relaxation.

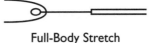

Full-Body Stretch

15. Become Your Own Best Friend Meditation

If you have more time, do the Become Your Own Best Friend Meditation that follows.

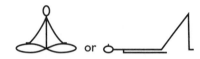

Become Your Own Best Friend Meditation

Cancer-Inspired Yoga Practice Overview

1. Mountain Pose. Silently repeat: *I am home in the here and now.*

2. Flower arms × 6. Inhale: *I am home.* Exhale: *Here and now.*

3. Albatross Sequence 1. Repeat the sequence × 4–6.

4. Warrior 1 variation. Inhale: *I am home.* Exhale: *Here and now.* Repeat × 6 on this side. Repeat on other side.

5. Warrior 1. Silently repeat × 3: *I am home in the here and now.*

6. Albatross Sequence 2. Repeat × 4.

7. Mantra *Ma* Sequence 1. Repeat × 4–6.

8a. Supine Twist with mantra *Vam.* Repeat × 6 on each side, alternating sides.

8b. Stay in Supine Twist for a few breaths. Repeat on other side.

9. Seated Forward Bend. Inhale: *I am home.* Exhale: *Here and now.* Repeat × 6 times. On final time stay for a few breaths.

10. Tortoise Pose. Stay for a few breaths. To work more gently skip this pose or do a Seated Forward Bend.

11. Mantra *Ma* Sequence 2. Repeat × 4–6.

12. Bridge Pose with arm movements. Inhale: *I am home.* Exhale: *Here and now.* Repeat × 6. Stay for a few breaths the final time.

13. Knees-to-Chest Pose. Rest here for a few breaths. Silently repeat × 3: *I am home in the here and now.*

14. Full-Body Stretch. Stay for a few breaths. *If short of time, finish here with a few minutes of relaxation.*

15. Become Your Own Best Friend Meditation.

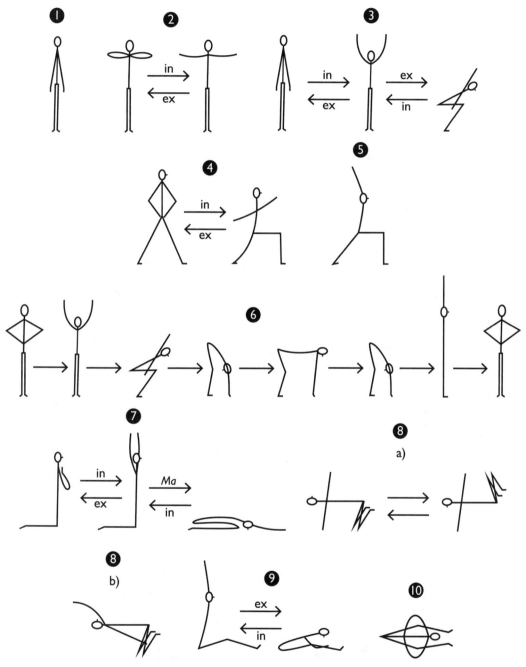

Cancer-Inspired Yoga Practice Overview

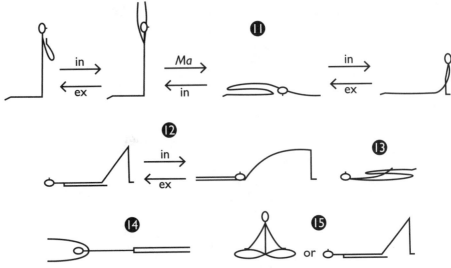

Cancer-Inspired Yoga Practice Overview (continued)

<hr>

MEDITATION
Become Your Own Best Friend

The zodiac sign Cancer is known as the mother sign, with a strong desire to nurture and nourish others. In this meditation we learn how to connect with our own inner loving, nurturing self. By cultivating good self-care in this way, we build up self-confidence and the resilience to cope with the ups and downs of life.

How do you talk to yourself when you mess up or life takes a wrong turn? Often at these difficult times our inner critic takes over, and many of us speak to ourselves in a manner that we would never dream of speaking to a friend.

As we journey through life, even though many of the events that occur in life are beyond our control, we can still consciously decide to cultivate a loving and compassionate attitude toward ourselves. This meditation teaches you to show the same compassion to yourself that you would show to a friend in need.

The meditation can be done sitting, lying, or as a walking meditation. If you choose to walk and meditate, you can either walk a fixed circuit, inside or out, or do the meditation while out on a walk. If you are outside, make sure you're aware of hazards such as traffic. Allow 10 to 15 minutes.

To begin the meditation, choose a minor problem that you are currently struggling with. Don't choose the biggest difficulty in your life; just choose something that's reasonably manageable. Then spend a few minutes turning this problem over in your head. As you do so, be aware of how you are feeling, both physically and emotionally. Notice any tension that arises in your body. Observe your internal dialogue and how you are speaking to yourself. Keep a background awareness of the natural flow of your breath.

Next imagine that rather than you, it is a close friend who is struggling with this problem. What advice, as a kind, caring friend, would you give to him or her? Notice your tone of voice, the kindness and affection you show them, and your understanding and empathy. What differences are there between the way you respond to your friend and the way you treat yourself when faced with the same dilemma?

Let go of the image of your friend. Notice how you are feeling now. Be aware of the natural flow of your breath.

Now, see if you can conjure up an image of what your ideal compassionate friend would be like. What qualities does this person have? It might be someone you know, someone you admire, or just an imaginary person. Choose someone who makes you feel safe, cared for, nurtured, and loved. Someone who would be there for you no matter what and who accepts you as you are and loves you unconditionally.

What would this person say if you were to share your problem with them? What advice would they give you? How would they respond to you? What wisdom would they impart to you regarding this difficulty? What action would they advise you to take? Allow yourself to feel loved, nurtured, and cared for by this person. Allow yourself to ask for what you need from them.

When you feel ready, thank this person for their love and guidance, give them a hug if you wish, and then let them go. Remember that contained within you are all the qualities that you admire in this ideal best friend. Whenever you choose, you can picture this person, and access the same kind, loving, wise, compassionate qualities within yourself.

Once again notice how you are feeling. Notice any physical sensations. Become aware of the natural flow of the breath. If you are sitting or lying, notice where your body is in contact with the floor or your support. If you are walking, become aware of the contact your feet are making with the earth with each step.

To conclude this meditation, spend a few moments considering what insights or wisdom you have gained from it. If you want to, write them down. If it feels right, give yourself a big, loving hug. Congratulate yourself for doing this meditation. Resolve to take this compassionate attitude back in to your everyday life and to be your own best friend today.

Cancer-Inspired Meditation Questions

See chapter 1 for guidance on how to use the meditation questions. The theme is "coming home to yourself."

- What is my recipe for a happy home?
- What do I need to make me feel at home?
  - What makes me feel ill at ease and disconnected?
- If I were to create a place of sanctuary, what would it be like? (Use all five senses to describe it: sight, smell, touch, taste, and feel.)
- Who makes me feel warm, safe, secure, and at home?
  - What qualities would my ideal loving and supportive friend have?
- What self-soothing techniques would I recommend to a friend who was feeling down or anxious?
- How does my ability to care for others compare with my ability to show good self-care to myself?
  - How would taking better care of myself make me more loving and caring toward others?
- Which yoga poses help me feel nurtured, nourished, and cared for?
  - Which meditation practices do the same?
  - What other activities help me feel, safe, secure, at ease, happy, and at home?

CHAPTER 8

Develop Fierce Confidence

♌

Leo

July 22–August 22

Connect with your powerful Sun self and radiate your light out into the world.

Yoga helps you stand tall and find the courage in your heart to follow your true path in life. Sometimes yoga is quiet and reflective, and at other times it prompts you to roar like a lion and to defend what you believe in. The reflective side of your yoga practice puts you in touch with what is true for you, whereas the active side of your practice requires you to give voice to that truth—and this is your lion's roar.

On the night of his enlightenment the Buddha sat under a tree and resolved to stay put until he reached the state of enlightenment. A long night followed, during which he was plagued by self-doubt manifesting as demons that tormented him. However, despite all that the demons threw at him, he stuck to his resolve and remained seated. Finally, in desperation the deity Mara appeared and challenged his very right to sit on that spot. The Buddha called upon the goddess of the earth, Prithivi, to bear witness to his right to take the one seat in recognition of his virtuous conduct, discipline, and spiritual practice perfected over many lifetimes. Grounded in the certainty of the earth's support, he roared like a lion and the demons evaporated.

Like the Buddha, we will all be challenged at times and our authority questioned. And like the Buddha, sometimes we will have to roar like a lion and declare our right to take the one seat. If you are a dedicated practitioner who has pursued a discipline over many years, then you have earned the right to stand up and make your voice heard. When you act as if you are prepared to stand up and fight, people will sense your mettle, and more often than not you won't be required to fight.

Yoga puts fire in your belly and a determination to make your voice heard above the noise. Whether you are teaching a yoga class, giving a presentation, writing a dissertation, or simply expressing a heartfelt view, consciously take the one seat. Own your expertise and assert your right to radiate your light out into the world. Imagine a golden crown upon your head as you to step into your own authority. Be the sun at the center of your own circle.

Confidence in your own abilities, a sense of your own authority, and the freedom of yoga can only be found through following a gentle discipline and a commitment to regular practice (*abhyasa*). Commitment for you might be honoring your intention to do five minutes of yoga a day and sticking to that. In practice this means every day, rain or shine, you show up. Whether you feel like doing yoga or not, you step onto your mat and do some yoga.

At times it takes courage to step onto your mat and face the crescendo of raw emotions that you are feeling. It may feel like there is no escape as you are brought face to face with your deepest self. It pays to have the courage to stay at the center of the circle and let the waves of emotions wash over you, even if it's only for five minutes at a time. This showing up and doing your yoga, whether you feel like it or not, is what the Buddha called "taking the one seat."[33]

The gentle discipline that you cultivate through your yoga practice will stand you in good stead in life. Courage is not the absence of fear; it is the judgment that something else is more important. And remember, you don't have to go it alone. At the heart of a lion pride is a closed sisterhood of female adults; they work cooperatively together, both in hunting and looking after their young. When we work collectively with others, we are stronger and can achieve more than when we work alone. So get together with other like minds and roar together in orchestrated chorus!

---

33. Jack Kornfield, *A Path with Heart* (London: Ebury Press, 2002), 35.

Yoga Inspired by Leo

Leo is a positive, fiery sign ruled by the Sun. Its key words are *creatively* and *joyfully*. Whereas our previous sign, Cancer, was traditionally associated with the mother, for Leo it is the father. The parts of the body that are associated with Leo are the heart and the spine. The sign has a regal nature, reflected in its favored royal colors, which are scarlet and gold.

In the Leo-inspired yoga practice that follows, we aim to build fierce, unshakeable confidence in tandem with a compassionate, loving heart. We draw our inspiration in this practice from the strength and courage of a lion as well as the lioness's ability to cooperate lovingly with other lionesses in her pride. Our intention to build a strength that is tempered by love is encapsulated in our affirmation for the practice, which is: *My strength is powered by love.*

Leo's rulership by the Sun is celebrated in this practice by including energizing, revitalizing sun imagery. We visualize a sun, radiating warmth and energy at the solar plexus chakra (*manipura*), and we use the empowering seed mantra *Ram*, which is associated with this chakra. This is our lion's roar. We temper this fierceness by including the compassionate seed mantra *Yam*, associated with the heart chakra (*anahata*). Stability is created and our connection to the earth strengthened by chanting the seed mantra *Lam*, which is associated with the earthy root chakra (*muladhara*).

We include flowing yoga sequences (*vinyasas*), incorporating yoga poses such as Chair Pose (*Utkatasana*) and modified press-ups to build up mental and physical strength. We also include the playfully fierce Lion Pose (*Simhasana*).

Leo-Inspired Yoga Practice

This yoga practice is inspired by the sign Leo, and it's suitable for everyone regardless of their sign. It's the go-to yoga practice whenever you need to be nurtured and empowered. It is centering, energizing, and uplifting, and it creates stability. It releases tension and blocked energy. It is a grounding, sunny, strengthening practice that increases confidence and courage.

The affirmation we use in the practice is *My strength is powered by love.* It can be shortened and coordinated with the breath:

Inhale: Strength

Exhale: Love

Allow 20 to 30 minutes.

1. Seated Sun visualization

Find yourself a comfortable, erect seated position. Picture in your mind's eye the Sun symbol, which is a dot within a circle. Then imagine that you are drawing a circle of light around yourself. Picture yourself as the Sun at the center of this circle. Now picture a sun, at your solar plexus, radiating light and warmth around your body. Silently repeat this affirmation three times: *My strength is powered by love.*

Seated Sun visualization

2. Bend and straighten warm-up

Take the legs 2 to 3 feet apart and turn the toes slightly out. Take the arms out to the sides at shoulder height, palms facing downward. On your next exhale, bend the knees and lower the arms. Inhale and return to the starting position. You can silently coordinate the breath and movement with the affirmation. Inhale and affirm, *Strength*. Exhale and affirm, *Love*. Repeat 6 times.

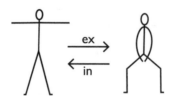

Bend and straighten warm-up

3. Lion Pose (Simhasana) *standing*

Take your legs 2 to 3 feet apart and turn the toes slightly out. Bend your arms and make a tight fist with your hands. Screw up your face, eyes shut tight. Exhaling, bend the knees, lean forward slightly, open your mouth wide, and stretch out your tongue, making a *ha* sound as you expel the breath; at the same time open your eyes wide and spread your fingers wide. Inhaling, straighten the legs and come back to the starting position with clenched fists. Repeat 4 times.

Lion Pose standing

4. *Dynamic Horse Pose* (**Vatayanasana**) *variation*

With legs 2 to 3 feet apart and toes turned slightly out, take both arms out to the side and above your head, bringing the hands together. Exhale, bend the knees as if you were sitting down on a high stool, and bring the hands to the heart. Inhaling, straighten the legs, taking arms out to the side and up above the head, back to the starting position. You can silently coordinate the breath and movement with the affirmation. Inhale and affirm, *Strength*. Exhale and affirm, *Love*. Repeat 6 times. On the final time stay for a few breaths in Horse Pose.

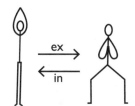

Dynamic Horse Pose variation

5. **Ram-Yam-Lam** *Sequence*

Stand tall, feet parallel and about hip width apart, with hands resting on the solar plexus. Inhale and take the arms out to the sides. On the exhale, chant *Ram* (pronounced *rum*), as you bring your hands back to the solar plexus. Inhale, taking the arms overhead. Exhale, lowering the arms and crossing the hands to the heart, as you chant *Yam* (pronounced *yum*). Inhale, taking the arms overhead. Exhale, coming into a Standing Forward Bend (*Uttanasana*) and chanting *Lam* (pronounced *lum*). Inhale, coming back up to standing and taking both arms up above the head. Exhale, lowering the hands back to the solar plexus. Repeat the sequence 3 more times.

Ram-Yam-Lam Sequence

6. Strengthening Salute to the Sun (Surya Namaskar *variation*)
Repeat 2 to 4 rounds of the following sequence:

6a. Mountain Pose (Tadasana) *with Sun visualization*
Stand in Mountain Pose (*Tadasana*) with your hands in Prayer Position (*Namaste*). In your mind's eye visualize the Sun in the sky. Now picture a warm, glowing sun at your solar plexus, radiating warmth and light, and keep this image in mind as you perform the Salute to the Sun (*Surya Namaskar*) variation.

Mountain Pose with Sun visualization

6b. Chair Pose (Utkatasana)
Stand tall, feet hip width apart and both arms above your head. Bend your knees and lower your bottom as if to sit down on a high stool. Keep the ears between the arms and don't round the upper back. Imagine that your hips are being pulled downward and everything above the waist is reaching skyward. Stay for a few breaths.

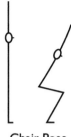

Chair Pose

6c. *Standing Forward Bend* (Uttanasana)

From Chair Pose (*Utkatasana*) allow your body to melt down into a Standing Forward Bend (*Uttanasana*). Then bend the knees and arch the back, and come back down into the forward bend.

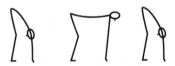

Standing Forward Bend

6d. *Plank Pose* (Chaturanga Dandasana)

Step the legs back, one at a time, into Plank Pose (*Chaturanga Dandasana*), holding the whole body in one long line.

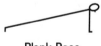

Plank Pose

6e. *Plank Pose* (Chaturanga Dandasana) *into Half Press-Ups*

From Plank Pose (*Chaturanga Dandasana*) lower the knees to the floor into a half press-up position. Do 4 press-ups, keeping the torso and thighs in one long line. (For a stronger version keep the legs straight and do full press-ups).

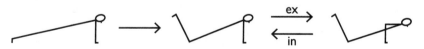

Plank Pose into Half Press-Ups

6f. *Plank Pose* (Chaturanga Dandasana) *into Child's Pose* (Balasana)

From Plank Pose (*Chaturanga Dandasana*) drop the knees to the floor, sitting back into Child's Pose (*Balasana*), and rest here for a few breaths.

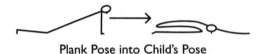

Plank Pose into Child's Pose

6g. *Child's Pose* (Balasana) *into Upward-Facing Dog Pose* (Urdhva Mukha Svanasana)

From Child's Pose (*Balasana*) come into Upward-Facing Dog Pose (*Urdhva Mukha Svanasana*).

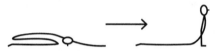

Child's Pose into Upward-Facing Dog Pose

6h. *Downward-Facing Dog Pose* (Adho Mukha Svanasana)

From Upward-Facing Dog Pose (*Urdhva Mukha Svanasana*) turn the toes under and swing back into a Downward-Facing Dog Pose (*Adho Mukha Svanasana*). Stay for a few breaths in the pose.

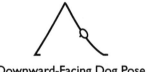

Downward-Facing Dog Pose

6i. *Lunge Pose* (Anjaneyasana)

From Downward-Facing Dog Pose (*Adho Mukha Svanasana*) bring your right foot forward into Lunge Pose (*Anjaneyasana*).

Lunge Pose

6j. *Standing Forward Bend (Uttanasana)*

Bring the back foot forward coming into a Standing Forward Bend (*Uttanasana*). Bend the knees and arch the back. Come back into the Standing Forward Bend and stay for a few breaths.

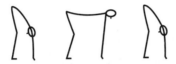

Standing Forward Bend

6k. *Mountain Pose* (Tadasana) *with Sun visualization*

From the Forward Bend, sweep the arms out to the sides and up above the head, coming back up to standing. Lower the hands back into the prayer position (*Namaste*) and rest here for a few breaths. As you rest, picture in your mind's eye, the Sun rising in the sky. And then picture a warm, glowing sun at your solar plexus; radiating warmth and light; and keep this image in mind as you perform another round of the Salute to the Sun. *Finish here or move on to step 7.*

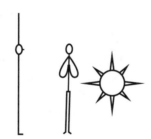

Mountain Pose with Sun visualization

7. *Universal Wind-Down Routine*

Conclude with the Universal Wind-Down Routine in chapter 1.

8. *Chakra Seed Mantra Meditation*

Do the Chakra Seed Mantra Meditation, which can be found on page 30, or if time allows, do the following Create Your Own Solar Mandala Meditation (if you are going for this option, make sure that you have paper and colored pens on hand).

Leo-Inspired Yoga Practice Overview

1. Seated Sun visualization.

2. Bend and straighten warm-up × 6.

3. Lion Pose × 4.

4. Dynamic Horse Pose × 6.

5. *Ram-Yam-Lam* Sequence × 4 rounds.

6. Strengthening Salute to the Sun × 2–4. *Finish here or move on to step 7.*

7. Universal Wind-Down Routine.

8. Chakra Seed Mantra Meditation (optional).

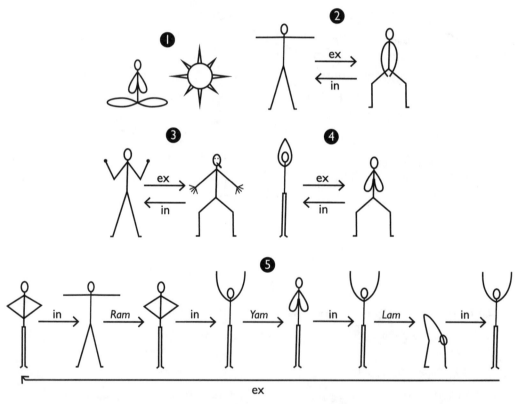

Leo-Inspired Yoga Practice Overview

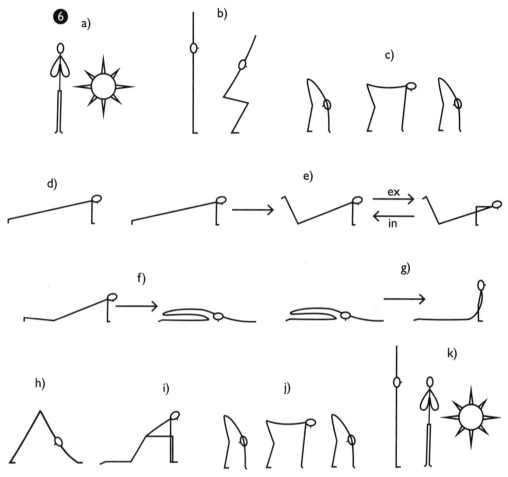

Leo-Inspired Yoga Practice Overview (continued)

MEDITATION

Create Your Own Solar Mandala

People of all zodiac signs can benefit from doing this meditation, but I've chosen it for the Leo chapter because Leo is ruled by the Sun, and this meditation helps us to connect with our powerful Sun energy, and use this "solar power" to create a life we love.

Mandala is the Sanskrit word for "circle." Hindus and Buddhists create mandalas that are complex and beautiful visual depictions of the universe. The mandala represents sacred or consecrated space. A deity is often to be found at the center of a mandala, surrounded by her or his kingdom.[34]

In this exercise you are going to create two mandalas. In the first you will make a depiction of your life as it *actually* is now. In the second you will create a mandala of your life as you would like it to be.

You will need two big sheets of plain paper and colored pens (or crayons, chalk, etc.). If you do not have these materials, you can make do with whatever paper and pens are available to you. Or if you prefer, you can do the exercise digitally. No artistic ability is necessary, and it doesn't matter how "messy" or unrealistic your depictions are! Adopt a meditative, playful attitude and enjoy the process of discovering something new about yourself.

This exercise will help you gain a clear, non-judgmental perspective on your life as it is now. It will also help you clarify any changes that you need to make in order to create a life that you love.

Find yourself a place where you will be undisturbed for 10 to 20 minutes. You can either sit at a table to draw or sit on the floor.

Start the meditation by spending a few minutes grounding and centering yourself. Have an erect posture, close your eyes, let go of unnecessary tension, and connect with the natural flow of your breath. Be aware of any thoughts and feelings that are arising. Aim to maintain this centered and meditative awareness throughout the exercise.

Step One

Take one of your sheets of paper and draw a big circle on it, either freehand or using a big plate or bowl. This circle represents the mandala of your life as it is now.

Sit quietly for a few breaths with your eyes closed and imagine what your life, as it is now, would look like as a circular mandala. Where do you see yourself on this mandala of your life? Are you at the center, to the side, up above, or down below? Open your eyes and draw yourself onto your mandala (or if you don't think you can draw, write your name in a color).

---

34. Simmer-Brown, *Dakini's Warm Breath*, 117.

Close your eyes again and get back in touch with the flow of your breath. Picture your life as it is now. Who else do you see in your circle? Now draw or write them onto your mandala.

What else do you want to add to your mandala? How do you spend your time and your energy? What is difficult and what brings you joy? Don't judge your life; simply try to create an honest, accurate picture of it as it is now.

Once you have finished, spend a few minutes looking at and meditating upon the mandala that you have created of your life as it is now. Then close your eyes. How do you feel now? What have you learned about yourself and your life?

Part of yoga is about having the courage and honesty to see things as they really are in the present moment. It is not about taking flight from reality. Yoga gives us the insight to see reality with crystal clearness. The actuality of how things are is our starting point. It's from this real place, with firm foundations, rooted in the earth and reality, that change is possible. Yoga also gives us the freedom and the space to dream the life that we would like to live, and this is what you are going to do with your second mandala.

Step Two

Take your second sheet of paper and draw a big circle on it. This is the circle of your life as you would like it to be.

Close your eyes and get back in touch with the natural flow of your breath. Notice how your body feels. Drop your awareness down to your solar plexus and imagine a radiant sun there.

This time picture yourself placed at the center of your mandala. You are like the Sun at the center of the solar system. Imagine yourself at the center, sitting on a throne; notice how grandly you are dressed. Open your eyes and draw or write yourself into the center of your mandala.

Close your eyes again and picture your own personal solar mandala. You are the sun at the center of your solar system. Who would you like to have close by you at the center of your circle? Now draw your chosen loved ones onto your mandala.

Close your eyes again. What else do you want to include in your dream life? How do you spend your time? What work do you do? What do you do in your spare time for fun? What's important to you?

Take up your pen again and complete your mandala, adding any details that you wish to create a picture of the life that you would love to live.

Feast your eyes upon the mandala that you have created. Compare it to the first mandala depicting your life as it is now. How do the two compare? How does it feel to place yourself like the Sun at the center of your mandala? Are you used to placing yourself at the center, or do you usually place yourself at the periphery of your life? What have you learned from this exercise? Are there any changes that you would like to make in your life? Is there a small step that you could take soon to make your dream life become a reality? Resolve to enjoy to the fullest all the good things about your life as it is now, while taking the steps necessary to create the change you dream of to create more beauty and joy in your life.

Leo-Inspired Meditation Questions

See chapter 1 for guidance on how to use the meditation questions. The Leo theme is "building confidence and unshakeable self-belief."

- How do I feel about the talents I have been endowed with?
  - Do I play down my talents for fear of appearing immodest?
- What am I passionate about?
    - Has following this passion led me to be an expert in my field?
    - How comfortable am I with owning this expertise and sharing it with others?
- How do I feel about authority—both my own and other people's?
    - Am I prepared to stand up for myself when others unfairly challenge my authority?
    - Am I able to confidently "take the one seat" and give voice to informed opinions?
- In what ways does perfectionism hold me back from reaching my full potential and gaining recognition for my achievements?
- What ideas do I have for collaborating and cooperating with others to work toward a shared vision?
- How do I support others to step into their authority and to find their own voice?

    – What ideas do I have for mentoring someone less experienced than me?

    – Am I able to listen to and learn from others?

    – Am I able to praise and affirm both myself and others?

- Which aspects of yoga do I find helpful for improving my self-confidence and developing an unshakeable belief in myself?

CHAPTER 9

Discover Your
Radiant Authentic Self

♍
Virgo

August 22–September 22

Find purity by honoring who you truly are.

Our yoga practice brings us face to face with our authentic self. When you truly know who you are, it becomes easier to bat away false projections and assumptions that others might make about you. The harvest of our yoga practice is uncovering a radiant authentic self within.

Purity (*sauca*) is one of the observances, or the personal disciplines, that make up the second of Patanjali's eight limbs of yoga. Yoga has a purifying, cleansing effect on a mental, physical, and emotional level. The yoga asanas, coordinated with the breathing, improve circulation and flush out toxins in our system. Deep relaxation allows the body to repair and renew itself.

However, the concept of purity can be a double-edged sword. One trap that we can fall into is to become obsessed with self-purification. Some yoga teachers exacerbate this tendency in their students by pushing the idea that we are all impure and need to follow extreme exercise routines and diets, including purging, to detoxify ourselves. Purity shouldn't become a stick to beat yourself with.

To avoid these pitfalls, it's important to choose a teacher who makes you feel good about yourself and allows you to be who you are. Don't stick with a teacher or organization that makes you feel bad about yourself. Although it can be motivating to have a teacher who gets you to push your boundaries, run a mile from one who makes you feel small and not good enough. There are so many good teachers and yoga groups out there, so use your intuition, inner wisdom, and bullshit filter to find one who is right for you.

Another trap we can fall into is trying to create a bubble of purity for ourselves. If you find yourself getting caught up in this trap, then try widening the lens, and rather than focusing exclusively on yourself, concentrate on working toward creating a purer, cleaner, healthier planet for everyone. The benefits of yoga's purifying practices are multiplied when combined with action to protect and purify the planet. Yoga is union, and as human beings, we are united by our dependence upon the earth for clean air, food, and water. At the same time remember to counterbalance your environmental campaigning with a mindful enjoyment of the beauty and bounty that this planet has to offer.

A commonly held belief in spiritually minded circles is if you want to change the world, then first change yourself. The idea is that the problem is with you and your attitude, rather than with the world around you. However, it's worth acknowledging that in reality there are systems in place that are discriminatory. The question we must ask is whether meditation alone is enough to overturn racism, sexism, homophobia, inequality, and so on. It's important that alongside our personal development work, we speak up, protest, and canvas for change.

Honoring who you are is purity. Demonizing people because of their difference is impurity. One of the beauties of the internet is that the usual gatekeepers are bypassed, so nowadays we see a much more diverse range of people depicted doing yoga. Whatever your age, color, gender, class, or sexual orientation, yoga will welcome you onto the mat. Embracing diversity is purity.

Purity is not a destination; it's a way of being. The beauty of yoga is that we experience ourselves from the inside out, rather than responding to the gaze of others and how they view us from the outside. Perhaps for the first time, we are comfortable in our own skin. This inner confidence helps us bat away projections from others who tell us that we are impure or not good enough. Yoga's inner journey helps us uncover what is true and pure within: our radiant authentic self.

Yoga Inspired by Virgo

Virgo is a mutable, earthy sign ruled by Mercury. The symbol for Virgo is a young woman with an ear of corn in her hand and a child in her lap. In Sanskrit she was known as *Kanya*, meaning virgin or maiden.[35] The Romans identified her with Ceres, Mother of the Corn, and Virgo's connection with food is reinforced by being known as the ruler of the digestive system. In the Northern Hemisphere Virgo's dates correspond with the harvest being brought in. She symbolizes fertility and purity.

The Virgo sign is also known for perfectionism, fastidiousness, and paying attention to small details. Whereas Pisces is concerned with infinite space, Virgo likes to put life under the microscope.

The Virgo symbol of feminine purity took me on an interesting path of study, which led me to discover more about Hindu attitudes to women and purity. The *Stridharma-paddhati* is a medieval Hindu text devoted to the subject of woman's nature and her appropriate duties. It states that owing to the process of menstruation and childbirth, women are considered innately impure and by nature sinful, and consequently they were forbidden from studying the sacred texts or hearing or reciting mantras. It states that a woman is not allowed to offer *puja* (worship) herself; her husband or priest must do it for her. However, there is also good evidence that in ancient times, previous to these restrictions, girls undertook spiritual initiation rites and were educated with boys.[36] Although this subject fascinates me, it's not within the scope of this book to go into it in more depth, but it does give us some clues to pursue if we want to find out more about women's notable absence from the history of yoga.

It is revealing to study the Virgo and Scorpio glyphs. Both have the same M-shaped structure, but Virgo has a serpent added to its glyph on the right side. According to astrologer Margaret Hone, this symbolizes woman's part in the Fall from grace in the biblical creation story (although, interestingly, in older creation myths the serpent was often said to represent wisdom and knowledge). Hone suggests that there were once

---

35. Walker, *The Woman's Dictionary of Symbols and Sacred Objects*, 295.

36. Lynn Teskey Denton, *Female Ascetics in Hinduism* (Albany: State University of New York Press, 2004), 24–28.

only ten signs, with Virgo and Scorpio being one sign. Then came the division into two and the insertion of Libra, and this created the twelve signs as we know them.[37]

I haven't been able to find further evidence to corroborate that Virgo and Scorpio were once one sign. However, I've found it a useful concept to allow me to explore the idea that on one side of Libra we have Virgo, an idealized version of feminine goodness, the virgin mother; and on the other side of Libra is Scorpio, the bad boy of the zodiac. Libra is the scales, and so we look to her to bring balance between these two gender polarities.

Let's come full circle and bring our Virgo theme back to yoga, turning to the three *gunas,* which in Tantric symbolism are the three "strands" of fate, colored white, red, and black. The three colors stood for "the divine female Prakriti," or Kali, in her triple aspects as Creator, Preserver, and Destroyer, or giver of birth, life, and death. The Virgin-Creator was *Sattva,* white; the Mother-Preserver was *Rajas,* red; the Crone-Destroyer was *Tamas,* black. Together they symbolized the cyclic succession of purity, passion, and darkness.[38]

We incorporate *Yoni Mudra* into one of our yoga sequences. A mudra is a hand gesture. The *Yoni Yantra* or triangle was known as the Primordial Image, representing the Great Mother as source of all life.[39]

In the practice we set the intention to cultivate the qualities of *sattva* in order to shed light on our radiant authentic self. We bring to the practice an awareness that when purity is conceived as an impossible-to-reach ideal imposed upon us from the outside, it can have a negative, detrimental influence. However, when it is arises from within, bathed in the pure light of self-awareness, it can be a health-enhancing, positive force. When in a state of contemplation, we come to rest in our true nature, which is true purity.

Virgo-Inspired Yoga Practice

Inspired by the zodiac sign Virgo, this practice has a devotional feel. It is deeply relaxing and grounding, and it will help you to access a deep source of strength and wisdom. It enables you to cultivate a sense of being comfortable in your own skin and to get in touch with the purity of your authentic self.

---

37. Hone, *The Modern Text-Book of Astrology,* 69.

38. Walker, *The Woman's Encyclopedia of Myths and Secrets,* 358.

39. Walker, *The Woman's Encyclopedia of Myths and Secrets,* 1098.

The affirmation we use in the practice is *The light within guides my way*. It can be shortened and coordinated with the breath:

Inhale: The light within

Exhale: Guides my way

Allow 20 to 30 minutes.

1. Easy Pose (Sukhasana) *with candle visualization*

Find yourself a comfortable seated position. Draw an imaginary circle of light around yourself. If it feels right, silently say, *I surround myself with love and light, and I am safe.* Bring your hands to your heart and visualize a candle flame burning steadily at the heart space. Then silently repeat your affirmation 3 times: *The light within guides my way.*

Ask to be given an image that symbolizes purity for you. If an image does not immediately come to mind, trust that at some point one will arise. If an image does arise, hold it in your heart as you do the practice.

If you wish, you can use the Universal Warm-Up Routine to prepare for this practice, or if you prefer, go straight on to step 2.

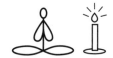

Easy Pose with candle visualization

2. Yoni Mudra Sequence

Do 6 rounds of this sequence:

2a. Mountain Pose (Tadasana)

Stand tall, feet parallel and about hip width apart. Make a triangle shape with the tips of your thumbs and index fingers (*Yoni Mudra*). Rest your *Yoni Mudra* hands on your lower abdomen with the triangle pointing downward.

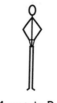

Mountain Pose

2b. *Raise arms forward*

Keeping your hands in *Yoni Mudra,* raise the arms forward and up to shoulder level.

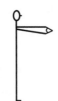

Raise arms forward

2c. *Arms out to the side*

Spread the arms out to the side.

Arms out to the side

2d. Yoni Mudra *overhead*

Take the arms overhead, bringing the hands back into an upward-facing triangle shape (*Yoni Mudra* overhead).

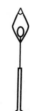

Yoni Mudra overhead

2e. *Standing Forward Bend* (Uttanasana) *variation*

Fold forward into a Standing Forward Bend (*Uttanasana*), bending the knees and sweeping the arms behind the back.

Standing Forward Bend variation

2f. Yoni Mudra *overhead*

Come back up to standing, taking the arms out to the sides and up above the head, bringing the hands back into *Yoni Mudra*.

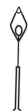

Yoni Mudra overhead

2g. *Mountain Pose with* Yoni Mudra

Lower the *Yoni Mudra* hands back to the starting position, with the downward-facing triangle resting on the lower abdomen. Repeat the *Yoni Mudra* sequence up to 5 more times.

Mountain Pose with *Yoni Mudra*

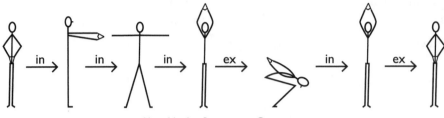

Yoni Mudra Sequence Overview

3. *Warrior Flow* (Virabhadrasana Vinyasa)

The following are steps for Warrior Flow (*Virabhadrasana Vinyasa*):

3a. *Warrior 2* (Virabhadrasana 2)

To start this flowing sequence, take the legs 2 to 3 feet apart, turning the left foot slightly in and right out. Bend the right knee. Take the arms out at shoulder height, palms facing down. Turn your head to look along your right arm. Stay here for a few breaths.

Warrior 2

3b. *Reverse Warrior Pose* (Virabhadrasana *variation*)

Keeping the right knee bent, lower the left hand to rest on the outside of the left thigh, reach the right arm up above the head and over to the left, and look up at the raised arm. Stay here for a few breaths.

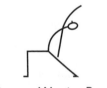

Reverse Warrior Pose

3c. Side-Angle Pose (Utthita Parsvakonasana)

Take the right forearm to rest on the right thigh (or for a stronger pose reach the hand down to the floor), taking the left arm over toward the left ear and keeping the chest rotating skyward. Stay here for a few breaths.

Repeat steps 3a, 3b, and 3c on the other side.

Side-Angle Pose

3d. Wide-Leg Standing Forward Bend Pose (Prasarita Padottanasana)

The legs are 2 to 3 feet apart, and the feet are parallel. Raise the arms out to the sides, just below shoulder height. Inhaling, hinge forward from the hip joints into a wide-leg forward bend. Bring the hands to the floor. For a gentler option bring the hands to rest on the legs or on raised blocks. Stay here for a few breaths, and then return to the starting position.

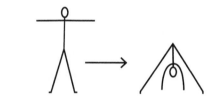

Wide-Leg Standing Forward Bend Pose

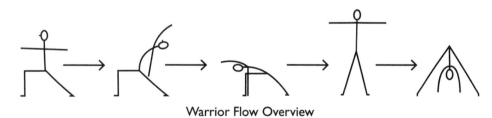

Warrior Flow Overview

4. Floor Salute to the Sun (Surya Namaskar variation)

The following are steps for the Floor Salute to the Sun (Surya Namaskar variation):

4a. Tall kneeling with visualization

Come to tall kneeling. Cross your hands at your heart and visualize a candle flame burning steadily at the heart space. Then silently repeat the affirmation 3 times: *The light within guides my way.*

Tall kneeling with visualization

4b. Tall kneeling into Child's Pose (Balasana)

Inhale, raising both arms above your head. Exhale, folding forward into Child's Pose (*Balasana*).

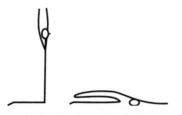

Tall kneeling into Child's Pose

4c. All fours into Downward-Facing Dog Pose (Adho Mukha Svanasana)

Inhale, coming onto all fours, and turn the toes under; exhaling, push into Downward-Facing Dog Pose (*Adho Mukha Svanasana*).

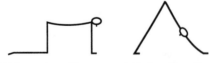

All fours into Downward-Facing Dog Pose

4d. Upward-Facing Dog (Urdhva Mukha Svanasana)

From Downward-Facing Dog Pose (*Adho Mukha Svanasana*), inhale, and swing into Upward-Facing Dog Pose (*Urdhva Mukha Svanasana*).

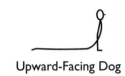

Upward-Facing Dog

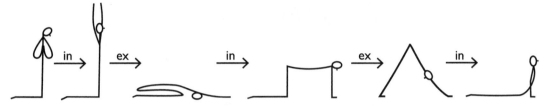

Floor Salute to the Sun Overview

4e. Perform sequence in reverse

Go back through the sequence in reverse order. Exhale into Downward-Facing Dog Pose (*Adho Mukha Svanasana*). Inhale back onto all fours. Exhale into Child's Pose (*Balasana*). Inhale, coming back up to tall kneeling and lifting arms above the head; exhale and return the hands to the heart. Repeat the sequence 4 to 6 times. (If you prefer, it's fine to ignore the breathing guidance that's given for this sequence. Take extra breaths if you need to. Never strain with the breathing.)

5. Bridge Pose (Setu Bandhasana) *with arm movements*

Lie on your back, knees bent and hip width apart. Inhaling, slowly peel the back from the floor and raise the arms above the head. Exhaling, lower the back to the floor and simultaneously lower the arms. Inhale and affirm, *The light within*. Exhale and affirm, *Guides my way*. Repeat 6 times, staying for a few breaths the final time.

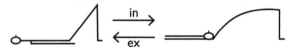

Bridge Pose with arm movements

6. Supine Twist (Jathara Parivrtti)

Lie on your back, knees bent, feet together, arms out to the sides at shoulder height, and palms facing down. Bring both knees onto your chest (for an easier pose keep both feet on the floor). Exhaling, lower both knees down toward the floor on the left and turn the head gently to the right. Inhale and return to center. With each exhale silently repeat the *bija* mantra *Vam* (pronounced *vum*). Allow your movements to be flowing and watery. Repeat 6 times on each side, alternating sides.

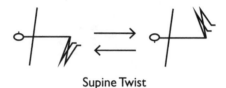

Supine Twist

7. Knees-to-Chest Pose (Apanasana) *into Leg Raises*

Bring both knees onto your chest. Inhale and straighten your legs vertically, heels toward the ceiling, taking your arms out to the side, just below shoulder height, palms facing up. Exhale and bring the knees back to the chest (*Apanasana*) and the hands back to the knees. Inhale and affirm, *The light within*. Exhale and affirm, *Guides my way*. Repeat 6 times.

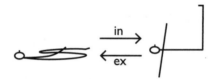

Knees-to-Chest Pose into Leg Raises

8. Seated visualization

Find yourself a comfortable position, either sitting or lying down. Draw an imaginary circle of light around yourself. If it feels right, silently say, *I surround myself with love and light, and I am safe*. Then bring your hands to your heart and visualize a candle flame burning steadily at the heart-space. Recall the image that symbolizes purity for you. If you have not yet received an image, ask once again to be given one. Then silently repeat the affirmation 3 times: *The light within guides my way*.

You could either end your practice here or go on to do the Pure World Visualization (see page 148) or the Chakra Seed Mantra Meditation (see page 30).

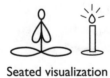

Seated visualization

Virgo-Inspired Yoga Practice Overview

1. Easy Pose with candle visualization.
2. *Yoni Mudra* Sequence × 6.
3. Warrior Flow.
4. Floor Salute to the Sun × 4–6.
5. Bridge Pose with arm movements × 6.
6. Supine Twist mantra *Vam* × 6 each side.
7. Knees-to-Chest Pose into Leg Raises × 6.
8. Seated visualization.

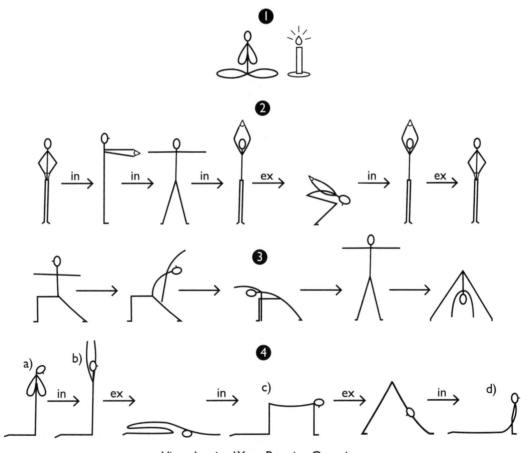

Virgo-Inspired Yoga Practice Overview

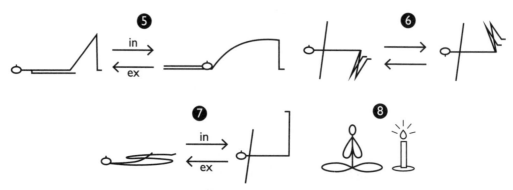

Virgo-Inspired Yoga Practice Overview (continued)

VISUALIZATION
Pure World

Virgo's element is earth, and its symbol represents purity, both of which are encapsulated in and have inspired this Pure World Visualization. The visualization enables us to widen our understanding of the yogic concept of purity (*sauca*) to include not only ourselves, but also the wider environment and the Earth itself.

Understandably, many of us are deeply concerned about the present state of the environment. Some of us react to this by burying our heads in the sand and end up feeling powerless to make the change that we desire. Others go into overdrive, and their activism can leave them feeling burned out and overwhelmed.

The Pure World Visualization offers us a way of acknowledging our concern for the environment while at the same time offering us hope through visualizing what a cleaned-up, pristine planet would be like. We also open our hearts to a deep love and gratitude toward our planet. This love and vision of hope for the world motivate and sustain us to take the actions needed to protect and purify the planet. The final stage of the meditation is when you step off the mat and make changes to try to create a cleaner, healthier planet.

The visualization can be done in any comfortable sitting or lying position. Allow 10 to 15 minutes.

We begin this meditation by recalling all the things that we love about planet Earth. What do you find beautiful about it? What brings you pleasure? What do you feel grateful for? Picture all the beauty and bounty that the Earth provides you with.

Spend a few minutes dwelling on any concerns you have for the planet. What environmental issues bother you? If you find yourself feeling overwhelmed by these concerns, just go back to observing your breathing and bodily sensations.

Now imagine that a miracle has happened, and our planet and its environment have been purified and made healthy and whole again. What does this purified planet look like? Imagine that you are breathing in pure, fresh air. The water in the streams and rivers is clear and clean and good enough to drink. The oceans have been cleaned up and are pristine again. The soil is fertile and full of nutrients needed for healthy plants, fruits, and vegetables. The natural world is thriving, and human beings are at one with their environment.

Picture yourself somewhere on this newly purified planet feeling safe and happy. Perhaps you are by a tranquil mountain pool with a waterfall. The water is clean enough to swim in. Or you might picture yourself high up on a mountain, enjoying the view and the pure, mountain air. Choose any place where you feel safe and at ease, and imagine yourself enjoying the beauty, tranquility, and purity of your surroundings. Be aware of sounds, sights, touch, and taste. Enjoy this clean, fresh environment with all your senses.

When you are ready, let go of the image of this idealized, pure world. Notice how you are feeling now; be aware of any thoughts or feelings that are arising. Allow yourself to feel whatever you are feeling, without judging or trying to fix it. Notice any bodily sensations; noting both areas of tension and relaxation. Observe the natural flow of your breath.

Once again, as we did at the start of this meditation, recall all the things that you love and appreciate about planet earth as it is now. Particularly, pay attention to all that is healthful about our planet. When you feel ready let this go and bring your awareness back to observing thoughts, feelings, bodily sensations, and the natural flow of your breath.

Then, if it feels right, consider whether there are any small steps that you could take to help to clean up our planet. What small, regular changes could you make that would help create a planet that is closer to the pure planet that you have envisioned? Remember that if we all make small changes in our behavior, it will have a big impact on our environment. After all, there is no planet B.

To conclude the meditation, become aware of where your body is in contact with the floor or your support. Feel your connection to the earth beneath you. Feel the space around you. Become aware of your surroundings, and when you are ready, carry on with your day.

Virgo-Inspired Meditation Questions

See chapter 1 for guidance on how to use meditation questions. The theme is "working with purity to create good health without and within."

- What does purity mean to me?
  - Complete the following sentence: "Purity is …"
- Which yoga techniques have I found helpful to cleanse and purify my system?
- There is a lot of money to be made from making people (especially women) feel "impure" and bad about themselves.
  - What negative messages of this sort have I internalized, and how do they play out in my life and the way I behave?
  - What do I find are the best ways to psychically protect myself from absorbing such negative projections?
  - How can I help others do the same so that they feel good about themselves too?
- Yoga teaches us to focus on how we feel on the inside, rather than obsessing about our outer appearance.
  - Which yoga techniques have I found help me to access a sense of being okay as I am?
  - Which other spiritual practices have helped me feel good about myself and comfortable in my own skin?
- If I were to picture a world where planet Earth has been cleaned up and is now pure and unpolluted again, what would it be like? What small steps could I take to make this dream become a reality?

CHAPTER 10

Creating Balance in Your Life

Libra

September 22–October 22

Learn to live harmoniously and in a state of equilibrium.

Our yoga practice opens us to the wisdom of the heart so that we can live harmoniously. The heart is the fulcrum that creates balance in our life. When we live from the heart, heaven and earth hold us in a state of equilibrium.

Yoga unites pairs of complementary opposites, such as passive and active, light and dark, chaos and order, left and right, soft and hard, pushing and yielding, and Sun and Moon energy. This reconciling of opposites creates the right conditions for balance and healing to occur.

The heart chakra (*anahata*) is the moderator between the material and the spiritual. It creates an energetic, figure eight–like pathway flowing between the lower, foundational chakras, and the higher, celestial ones. There are seven subtle energy centers (*chakras*) to be found within the body. There are three "lower" chakras below the heart, associated with material, earthly concerns, and three "higher" chakras above the heart associated with spiritual matters.

Many of us are initially drawn to yoga because we are hoping to impose order upon our chaotic lives. We long for a life that is harmonious, peaceful, and in balance. Yoga asanas, *pranayama*, relaxation, and meditation help restore balance to body and mind. They work at a deep, therapeutic level on the systems that enable us to maintain a healthy state of equilibrium. Yoga also calms the turbulent water of a troubled mind, restoring a more harmonious, peaceful state of being.

However, yoga is not a wall we build around a static state of harmony. Ideally, periods of peaceful repose are balanced with action to create a more harmonious world for everyone. We create balance in our life by making judgments and weighing one thing up against another. We put our lives on the scales and decide: yes, this is right, or no, this is wrong. When we remain silent about injustice, we may find temporary peace, but something inside of us dies. To be able to judge, we need a clear, all-seeing eye. To see clearly, we must keep our head, while at the same time viewing the situation through the lens of the heart.

Your inner state of balance is in relationship with and dependent upon your outer environment. There is an umbilical cord that connects you to the outside world through the air that you breathe, the food that you eat, and the water that you drink. Your health is intimately connected to the health of the planet. If the planet's ecosystem is out of balance, your system will be stressed too. When we work for the health of the planet, we work for our own health too.

Equilibrium is achieved through a dynamic exchange between our inner and the outer environment. This is referred to as homeostasis. Your body has an incredible wisdom and always attempts to maintain constant internal conditions regardless of the fluctuations in the outer environment. This dynamic balancing act ensures you stay healthy and, for that matter, alive.

Our yoga practice creates the right conditions for us to return to a neutral state of perfect equilibrium. This balanced state is one of total acceptance: life is as it is. We move in and out of this state of perfect peace. Yoga helps us get a perspective on our life. We learn to let go of striving to impose order upon the chaos of our life; all is held in the heart with love and compassion.

Yoga Inspired by Libra

The zodiac wheel is thought by some to symbolize the cycle of life, death, and rebirth. The first six signs of the zodiac, from Aries to Virgo, are considered to be more materially oriented, whereas the last six signs, from Libra to Pisces, are deemed more spiritual. So a journey around the wheel of the zodiac is an evolution from the material to the spiritual, which is in itself a form of yoga.[40] Whereas the first six signs were more outward looking, the second six signs are more inward looking, and this homeward journey back to the self commences with the sign Libra.

Libra is a cardinal air sign ruled by Venus. Its symbol is the weighing scales. The Sanskrit name for the sign of Libra was *Tula*, the Balance.[41] Libra was known as the astrological Lady of the Scales, and she represented the balancing process of karmic law.[42] The endocrine system, which maintains the body in a balanced state, is assigned to Libra. Libran colors are blues and pinks. Its metal is copper. Key words are *harmoniously* and *unitedly*.

Libra is the fulcrum balancing the material and spiritual world, reminding us that what is considered "lower" supports that which is above and that the two worlds are united by love. This is beautifully encapsulated in the equilibrium of the figure-eight glyph, the symbol of infinity, which is associated with Libra. This is mirrored in the body's chakra system, where the heart center balances the lower and higher chakras in a loving and compassionate way. It is this connection that inspired the Heart-Centered Balancing Meditation, which follows the yoga practice in this chapter.

Libra, like yoga, helps us balance pairs of opposites, such as Sun and Moon, light and dark, masculine and feminine, passive and active, pushing and yielding, and order and chaos. This reconciliation of pairs of opposites creates balance and healing. Libra encourages us to ask the question "How do we create balance in our yoga practice and in our life?"

Libra-Inspired Yoga Practice

The Libra-inspired yoga practice that follows balances and realigns the body and mind, both physically and energetically. It is calming and quietly energizing and has a centering effect. It soothes a restless mind, restoring balance and equanimity. The heart center

---

40. MacNeice, *Astrology*, 82.

41. Walker, *The Woman's Dictionary of Symbols and Sacred Objects*, 292.

42. Walker, *The Woman's Encyclopedia of Myths and Secrets*, 538.

chakra is gently opened, helping us develop a sense of love and compassion for ourselves and others.

The affirmation we use in the practice is *My heart balances all.* It can be coordinated with the breath:

Inhale: My heart balances all

Exhale: My heart balances all

Allow 20 to 30 minutes.

1. Centering Meditation

Find yourself a comfortable position lying down. Bring your awareness to the midline of your body; particularly, be aware of the entire length of your spine. Then take your awareness to the left side of your body. Explore how this side of your body feels, noticing any sensations that arise. Next take your awareness to the right side of your body. Notice how the two sides of the body compare. Is one side heavier, lighter, tighter, more relaxed?

Take your awareness back to the left side of your body. As you inhale, imagine that you are breathing into and energizing the left side; as you exhale, imagine that you are letting go of any tension in that side of the body. Inhale: energize. Exhale: relax. Repeat over several breaths. Before you change sides, notice how both sides of your body feel. Is there any difference between the side you have been breathing into and the other side? Then repeat on the right side of your body. Conclude by breathing into and out from both sides of the body. Inhale: energize. Exhale: relax.

Silently repeat this affirmation 3 times: *My heart balances all.*

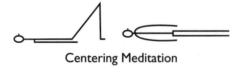

Centering Meditation

2. Cat Pose (Marjaryasana) *into* Cow Pose (Bitilasana)

Start on all fours. Exhaling, round the back up like an angry cat. Inhale into Cow Pose, arching the back, lifting the chest up and away from the belly, and looking up slightly.

Alternate between these two positions, rounding and arching the back, and repeat 8 times. (If you have a back problem, don't arch the back.)

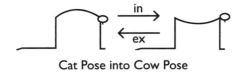

Cat Pose into Cow Pose

3. Cat Pose (Marjaryasana) *with leg movements*

Start on all fours. Exhaling, round the back and bring the left knee toward the head and the head toward the knee. Inhaling, take the left leg out behind you and in line with the torso. Repeat 6 times on this side and then repeat on the other side.

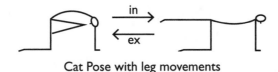

Cat Pose with leg movements

4. Tiger Pose (Vyaghrasana) *variation*

Start on all fours. Extend your straightened left leg out behind you, toes curled under and resting on the floor. Extend your right arm out along the floor in front of you, fingertips resting on the floor. Inhale to prepare. Exhale and raise the extended arm and leg up and in line with the torso. Keep the pelvis level. Stay in the pose, inhaling and stretching further. Exhaling, lower the arm and leg back to the starting position. Repeat 6 times on this side, staying for a few breaths in the pose on the final time. Repeat on the other side.

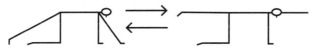

Tiger Pose variation

5. Tall kneeling to Child's Pose (Balasana), *single arms*

Come to tall kneeling. Raise your right arm above your head and place your left hand behind your back. Exhaling, fold forward into Child's Pose, keeping your left hand resting on your lower back. Inhale and come back up to the starting position. Repeat 3 times on this side and then 3 times on the other side.

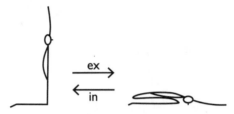

Tall kneeling to Child's Pose, single arms

6. Tall kneeling to Child's Pose (Balasana)

From tall kneeling, raise both arms above your head. Exhale, folding forward into Child's Pose. Silently repeat the affirmation *My heart balances all* on both the inhale and the exhale. Repeat the sequence 3 times.

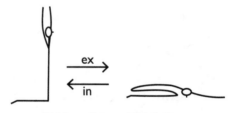

Tall kneeling to Child's Pose

7. Sitting Side Bend

Come into a cross-legged sitting position. Arms straight and out to the sides, fingertips resting lightly on the floor. Inhale, raising your right arm and stretching your torso over to the left. Exhale, lowering your arm to the starting position. Repeat 6 times on this same side, staying for a few breaths on the final time. Repeat on the other side.

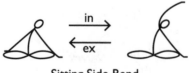

Sitting Side Bend

8. Gate Pose (Parighasana) *with arm movements*

Come to tall kneeling. Extend your left leg straight and out to the side. Rest your left hand on your left thigh. Your right arm is by your side. Inhale, raising your right arm above your head, and side-bend toward your left leg. Exhale, coming back to center and lowering your arm back to the side. Repeat 4 times, and on the final time stay a few breaths in the pose. Come back to center and then repeat on the other side.

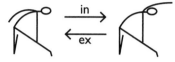

Gate Pose with arm movements

9. Gate Pose (Parighasana)

From tall kneeling, extend your left leg out to the side. Rest your left hand on your left thigh and take your right hand down to rest on the floor, in line with your right knee. Stretch your left arm over head to the right. Keep your torso rotating skyward. Stay here for a few breaths. Come back to center and then repeat on the other side.

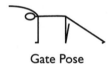

Gate Pose

10. Downward-Facing Dog Pose (Adho Mukha Svanasana) *with arm raises*

From all fours push up into Downward-Facing Dog (*Adho Mukha Svanasana*). Stay here for a few breaths. Then take your right hand to touch your right sitting bone. Repeat on the left side. Repeat 3 times on each side.

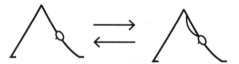

Downward-Facing Dog Pose with arm raises

11. Plank Pose (Chaturanga Dandasana) *into Side Plank Pose* (Vasisthasana)

From Downward-Facing Dog Pose (*Adho Mukha Svanasana*), lower yourself into Plank Pose (*Chaturanga Dandasana*), the whole body in one long line. Stay a few breaths here and then swivel to one side into Side Plank Pose (*Vasisthasana*). Stay a few breaths. Repeat on the other side.

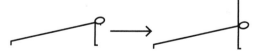

Plank Pose into Side Plank Pose

12. *Child's Pose* (Balasana) *into Upward-Facing Dog Pose* (Urdhva Mukha Svanasana)

From sitting kneeling, sit back into Child's Pose (*Balasana*), arms outstretched along the floor. Inhale and move forward into Upward-Facing Dog Pose (*Urdhva Mukha Svanasana*), arching your back and keeping your knees on the floor. Exhale back into Child's Pose. You can silently coordinate the breath with the affirmation. Inhale and affirm, *My heart balances all*. Exhale and affirm, *My heart balances all*. Repeat 6 times, as you move between the two poses.

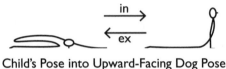

Child's Pose into Upward-Facing Dog Pose

13. *Heart Chakra Sequence*

Start in Child's Pose (*Balasana*), with forearms and hands on the floor just above your head. Inhale and come up to tall kneeling, taking arms above your head. Exhale and chant the mantra *Yam* (pronounced *yum*) as you cross your hands and place them on your heart. Inhale, raising the arms up above your head again. Exhale, coming back to Child's Pose. Repeat the sequence 6 times.

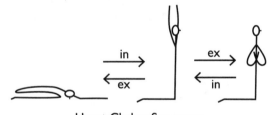

Heart Chakra Sequence

14. *Centering Meditation*

We end this session as we began it, with the Centering Meditation. Find yourself a comfortable position lying down. Bring your awareness to the midline of your body; particularly, be aware of the entire length of your spine. Then take your awareness to the left side of your body. Explore how this side of your body feels, noticing any sensations that arise. Next take your awareness to the right side of your body. Notice how the two sides of the body compare. Is one side heavier, lighter, tighter, more relaxed?

Take your awareness back to the left side of your body. As you inhale, imagine that you are breathing into and energizing the left side; as you exhale, imagine that you are letting go of any tension in that side of the body. Inhale: energize. Exhale: relax. Repeat over several breaths. Before you change sides, notice how both sides of your body feel. Is there any difference between the side you have been breathing into and the other side? Then repeat on the right side of your body. Conclude by breathing into and out from both sides of the body. Inhale: energize. Exhale: relax.

Then, silently repeat the affirmation 3 times: *My heart balances all.*

You can either finish your practice here or, if you have time, do the Heart-Centered Balancing Meditation that follows.

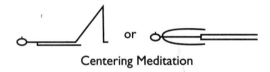

Centering Meditation

Libra-Inspired Yoga Practice Overview

1. Centering Meditation.

2. Cat Pose into Cow Pose × 8.

3. Cat Pose with leg movements × 6. Repeat on other side.

4. Tiger Pose × 6. On final time stay a few breaths. Repeat on other side.

5. Tall Kneeling to Child's Pose, single arms, × 3. Repeat on other side.

6. Tall Kneeling to Child's Pose × 3.

7. Sitting Side Bend × 6. On final time stay a few breaths. Repeat on other side.

8. Gate Pose with arm movements × 4. On final time stay a few breaths. Repeat on other side.

9. Gate Pose. Stay a few breaths. Repeat on other side.

10. Downward-Facing Dog Pose with arm raises × 3 on each side.

11. Plank Pose into Side Plank Pose. Repeat on other side.

12. Child's Pose into Upward-Facing Dog Pose × 6.

13. Heart Chakra Sequence × 6.

14. Centering Meditation.

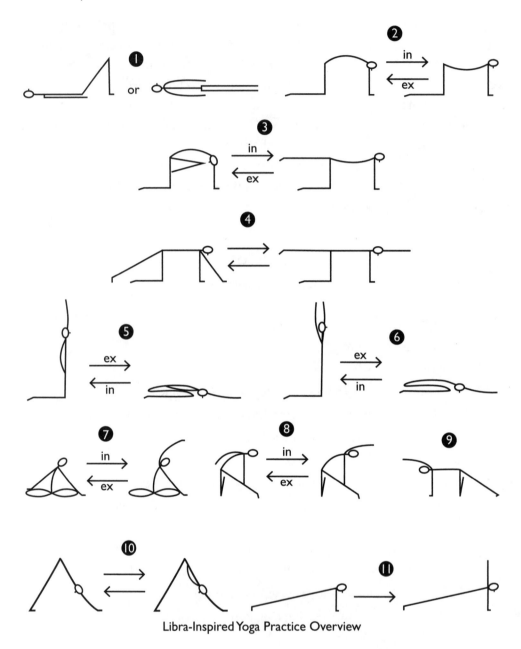

Libra-Inspired Yoga Practice Overview

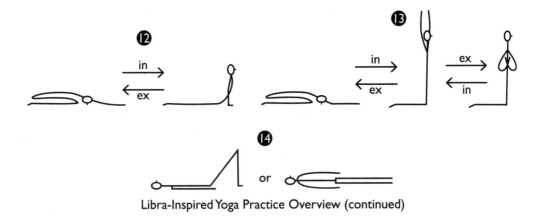

Libra-Inspired Yoga Practice Overview (continued)

<hr>

MEDITATION

Heart-Centered Balancing Meditation

This meditation teaches us to bring harmony and equilibrium on both a physical and spiritual level through learning to radiate love from our heart to the lower and higher chakras in our body. This ties in with the Libra theme, as within the zodiac Libra is the fulcrum balancing the material and spiritual world.

The chakras are a real treasure trove of inspiration, encompassing colors, mandalas, sounds, gemstone, gods and goddesses, planets, and so on. I hope this meditation whets your appetite to discover more about them. It's impossible to define exactly what the chakras are or to pinpoint exactly where they are located in the body. Personally, I favor the argument that the chakras are a poetic device that enables us to explore the body's subtle energy system. This poetic model, as opposed to a literal one, gives us the freedom to intuit where the chakras are in the body and to allow our imagination to run freely. For simplicity in this meditation I adhere to the seven-chakra system (see page 28).

When life feels out of kilter and chaotic, this meditation will help you regain a sense of order. It will help restore your equilibrium when you're feeling anxious, preoccupied, or overwhelmed. It enables you to surround your difficulties with love and compassion. It shifts stuck energy and entrenched patterns of behavior.

Allow 10 to 15 minutes.

Find yourself a comfortable sitting position, either on the floor or on a chair. Adopt a tall, erect, but relaxed posture. Notice which parts of the body are in contact with the floor or your support. Relax into this support and feel yourself held by the earth beneath you. Be aware of the space around your body and allow yourself to expand into this sense of spaciousness.

Become aware of the midline of the body; feel yourself symmetrically organized around this midline. Take your awareness from the base of your spine up to the crown of your head; sense a connection between the base of the spine and the earth below you, and the crown of the head and the sky above you. Feel yourself centered and aligned.

Now bring your awareness to your heart chakra (*anahata*). If you wish, you can place one hand on top of the other at the heart center. Engender a sense of love and compassion for yourself; feel this love radiating from the heart all around the body.

Now take your awareness to the three chakras below the heart. Begin at the root chakra (*muladhara*). It is said to be located in the pelvic floor area near the base of the spine. Then take your awareness up to the creation chakra (*svadhisthana*) in the lower belly, then up to the solar plexus chakra (*manipura*).

Imagine that the heart center is sending love and compassion to all these lower chakras. Feel the warm light of love radiating from the heart to your lower body.

Draw your awareness from the lower body back up to the heart. Then begin to explore the three chakras above the heart: the communication chakra (*vishuddha*) at the throat; the intuition chakra (*ajna*), located between the brows at the "third eye"; and the crown chakra (*sahasrara*), located in the space just above the crown of the head.

Come back to your heart center and imagine the heart sending love and compassion to all the three higher chakras. Feel the warm light of love radiating from the heart to your upper body.

Once again return your awareness to the heart, and this time picture the heart sending love and compassion to both the upper and lower body. Feel the warm rays of love and light emanating from the heart and radiating throughout the body.

Now picture an 8 shape. Imagine that your heart is at the center of the 8 shape, uniting the higher and lower chakras and powering a perpetual loop of energy circulating around the 8 shape. The figure eight is the symbol for infinity and originated in India.[43] When you feel ready, let go of the image.

It's important to ground yourself after working with the chakras. You can do this by bringing your awareness to the lower body, particularly noticing where the body is in contact with the floor or your support. Feel your connection to the earth beneath you.

Next bring the hands up to the heart and make a flower shape of them: the heels of the hands are together and the fingers spread like open petals. Slowly close the petal fingers until the hand resembles a flower in bud. Stay here for a few more breaths and then return the hands to rest in the lap or on the thighs. Resolve to take this loving, compassionate, heart-centered energy back into your everyday life and into the very next thing you do today.

Libra-Inspired Meditation Questions

See chapter 1 for guidance on how to use the meditation questions. The theme for Libra is "creating a balanced life."

- If I listened to my heart, how would I go about creating balance in my life?
- How does it feel when my life is in balance?
  - When my life is out of balance, what's different?
- How could I improve the balance between time spent doing things I love and time spent doing things I feel I ought to do?
- Who helps me to live in a balanced way?
  - Who throws me off balance?
- What is the best way to stay balanced when faced with stressful situations, people, or environments?
- If I were to imagine a world where peace and justice were available to everyone, what would it be like?
  - Are there any small steps I could take to bring this harmonious world a step closer?

---

43. Walker, *The Woman's Dictionary of Symbols and Sacred Objects*, 9.

- What would the world be like if our ecosystem were in balance?
  - How does environmental pollution impact on my own and others' health?
  - Are there any small steps I could take to improve the environment for myself and others?
- Which yoga techniques do I find help me stay grounded, centered, and balanced?

CHAPTER 11

Face Fear and Find Freedom

♏
Scorpio

October 22–November 22

Shine light into the darkness and transform suffering to joy.

Our lives are mandalas. Within the circle of our life are to be found sunshine and shadow, highs and lows, happiness and sadness, gains and losses, and birth and death. Your yoga practice is there for you even on the darkest of days and the longest of nights.

Yoga philosophy teaches that attachment (*raga*) and aversion (*dvesa*) cause us to suffer. Naturally, we want to cling to happiness and push away unhappiness. The nature of life is that everything changes. We all know this; we may on an intellectual level accept it, but the lived reality of change can be hard. Sometimes life, like a scorpion, has a sting in the tail.

The Bhagavad Gita tells us that whether we want to fight the battle of life or not, our karma will impel us to. Life can be scary sometimes, but if you practice yoga when things are going well and build strong foundations, you'll be better prepared to weather life's storms.

The Buddha encouraged his monks and nuns to go to the charnel ground to receive a lesson in impermanence by contemplating the body of someone who had recently died. The charnel ground is the place where the dead are cremated; it is a sacred space where the conditions are right for transforming fear into awakening. For present-day practitioners the charnel ground could be any situation that offers you the opportunity to transform fear into awakening. If old age scares you, then visiting a relative with dementia in a care home might be your charnel ground.

The gentle discipline of our yoga practice is to learn to turn toward unpleasant emotions, rather than push them away. The poet Rumi, in his much-quoted poem "The Guest House," said that you should welcome and "entertain" even negative emotions such as sorrow or depression, because they may be "clearing you out for some new delight." [44]

When we turn toward that which we fear most, we find much that needs composting, as well as hidden treasure. In yoga *apana* is the eliminative energy that helps rid our system of toxins and waste. The out-breath uses *apana* energy to eliminate and remove physical, mental, or emotional toxicity from body and mind.

A challenging yoga pose gives us the opportunity to rehearse staying present and focused despite mild physical discomfort and waves of strong emotions arising. We breathe in, and we feel what we are feeling in our body. We breathe out, letting go, or if we can't let go, we let it be. We notice when our mind has been carried away from the here and now by a story it is telling itself, and we gently return to the present moment.

We learn to recognize that each emotion resides as an echo somewhere in our body. We lovingly embrace the frustration that has tightened our shoulders, caress the fear that has locked up our diaphragm, and free the butterflies of anticipation that are fluttering around our chest. We breathe in, we breathe out. We take one breath at a time. Just this breath, just this moment. We quiet down so that we can hear the still, small voice of calm, which will guide us safely through the storm.

Yoga is a Full Moon on a dark, cold night. It is old brown leaves in autumn and new buds unfurling on the tree in spring. Yoga relaxation frees that which was hidden and bound in the subconscious. In dreamlike states, that which was concealed in cobwebbed

---

44. Rumi, "The Guest House," in *The Essential Rumi*, trans. Coleman Barks and John Moyne (San Francisco: Harper, 1997), 109.

corners of the mind is revealed and brought up into the light of our awareness. Into those dark spaces we shine a light of kind and loving attention.

Yoga Inspired by Scorpio

Scorpio is a fixed, negative water sign that is ruled by Mars. Its symbol is the scorpion, which in Sanskrit is *Vrischika*. It's a sexual sign, associated with the processes of birth, life, death, and rebirth. Its metal is iron, and its color deep red. The plants that Scorpio is associated with are those that sting or have thorns (such as brambles, nettles, and thistles) or the pungent and spicy ones (such as garlic and ginger). Key words are *passionately*, *secretively*, and *penetratingly*.

Scorpio is associated with endings and new beginnings. In the Northern Hemisphere its dates coincide with the transition from autumn to winter, and this may be where its association with death and decline arises from. The heavenly constellation of Scorpio presided over the Celtic festival of Samhain (Halloween) or the Feast of the Dead.[45] Scorpio invites us into the darkness, the place where life ends and new life begins.

The sting in the tail of Scorpio makes it one of the most challenging, and at the same time one of the most rewarding, signs to work with. To uncover the treasure buried within the sign we must move toward what scares us most, rather than avoiding it.

Our yoga practice can provide us with the stability to do the warrior work of approaching and befriending our fears. In the more challenging asanas, we learn how to lean into discomfort, finding our edge without leaping off it into full-blown pain. We also cultivate compassion for our struggles and difficulties, surrounding them with love and understanding. The eagle is another symbol associated with this sign, and our practice of yoga teaches us the eagle-like skill of rising above our everyday concerns and seeing the bigger picture. In this way we experience freedom.

Scorpio is also ruled by the dwarf planet Pluto, which gives a deep and mysterious aspect to the sign. Pluto is associated with that which is bound and hidden, such as the subconscious and the deepest recesses of the mind. It is known for its quick, forceful, eliminative, ejecting action, which in yoga we might relate to *apana*, which is the eliminative energy that helps rid our system of toxins and waste. Yogic techniques such as *kapalabhati*, in which we forcefully expel air from the lungs, correspond with this Plutonian eliminative action.

---

45. Walker, *The Woman's Dictionary of Symbols and Sacred Objects*, 294.

Scorpio-Inspired Yoga Practice

In the Scorpio-inspired yoga practice that follows, we use the *Ha* breath and the Lion Pose (*Simhasana*) for their cleansing, purifying, detoxifying effect and their ability to shift stuck or stagnant energy. The practice brushes away the cobwebs and opens the mind to fresh, new inspiration.

The affirmation we use in the practice is *Love surrounds all my feelings*. It can be coordinated with the breath:

> *Inhale:* Love surrounds
>
> *Exhale:* All my feelings

Allow 20 to 30 minutes.

1. Mountain Pose (Tadasana)

Stand tall, feet parallel and about hip width apart. Be aware of the contact between your feet and the earth beneath you. Imagine a string attached to the crown of your head, gently pulling you skyward; simultaneously, let your tailbone drop and feel your heels rooting down into the earth. Silently repeat the affirmation 3 times: *Love surrounds all my feelings.*

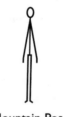

Mountain Pose

2. Ha *breath*

Stand in Mountain Pose (*Tadasana*). Inhale, taking both arms out to the side at just below shoulder height. Exhale, making a *Ha* sound as you bend the knees, lean slightly forward, and bring both hands to the belly. Return to the starting position on the inhale. Repeat 3 to 6 times.

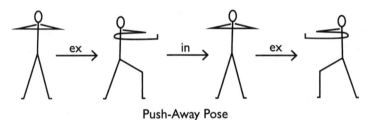

Ha breath

3. *Push-Away Pose*

Take your feet 2 to 3 feet apart, toes turned slightly out. Rest your fingertips lightly on your shoulders, elbows out to the sides. Exhaling, bend your right knee, take your left arm across your chest, and push the heel of your hand toward the right side of the room. Your torso stays facing forward. Inhale and come back to center. Repeat to the other side. Each time you exhale and push away, imagine that you are pushing away anything you wish to expel from your life. Repeat 6 times on each side, alternating sides.

Push-Away Pose

4. *Lion Pose* (Simhasana)

Keep the legs 2 to 3 feet apart, toes turned slightly out. Bend your arms and make a tight fist with your hands. Screw up your face, eyes shut tight. Exhale, bend the knees, lean slightly forward, and open your mouth wide as you stretch out your tongue, making a *Ha* sound as you expel the breath. At the same time open your eyes wide and spread your fingers wide. Inhaling, straighten the legs and come back to the starting position with clenched fists. Repeat 4 times.

Lion Pose

5. Dynamic Side Bend

Keep the legs 2 to 3 feet apart, toes turned slightly out and arms by your side. Inhale as you bend your right knee, and raise your left arm overhead into a side bend to the right. Exhaling, lower the arm and straighten the leg, returning to the starting position. You can silently coordinate the breath and movement with the affirmation. Inhale and affirm, *Love surrounds.* Exhale and affirm, *All my feelings.* Repeat 6 times on this same side, and on the final time stay for a few breaths in the side bend. Repeat on the other side.

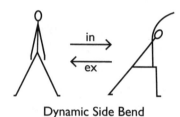

Dynamic Side Bend

6. Extended Side Angle Pose (Utthita Parsvakonasana)

Take the legs 3 to 4 feet apart and turn the right foot slightly in and left foot out. Bend the left knee. Take the arms out at shoulder height, palms facing down. From here bring your left forearm to rest on your bent left knee or bring your fingertips to rest on the floor just outside your left foot. Your right hand reaches up toward the sky or over toward your ear. Keep your chest rotating skyward. Stay for a few breaths.

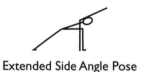

Extended Side Angle Pose

7. Wood-Chop Squat with Ha breathing

Stand with your feet parallel, shoulder width apart. Raise both arms above your head, fingertips touching. Bend your knees into a squat, keep your arms straight, and chop down, making a *Ha* sound on the out-breath. Inhale and come back to the starting position. Repeat 6 times.

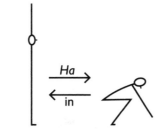

Wood Chop Squat with *Ha* breathing

8. *Half-Moon Pose* (Ardha Chandrasana)

Stand in Mountain Pose (*Tadasana*) sideways on your mat. Take the legs 3 to 4 feet apart and turn the right foot slightly in and the left foot out. Bend the left knee, take the arms out to the sides at shoulder height, palms facing forward. Bend your left knee and reach your left hand down to the floor just beyond your left foot (or onto a block). Shift your weight over your supporting leg and lift your right foot off the ground until the leg is horizontal to the floor, simultaneously rotating your chest skyward and raising your right arm until it is in line with your left arm. Stay for a few breaths. To come out of the pose, bend your left knee and lower the right foot back to the floor. Repeat on the other side. When you are learning this pose, try practicing with your back to a wall for support.

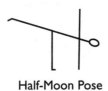

Half-Moon Pose

9. *Mountain Pose* (Tadasana) *into Chair Pose* (Utkatasana)

Stand in Mountain Pose (*Tadasana*), hands in Prayer Position, and silently repeat the affirmation 3 times: *Love surrounds all my feelings.* From Mountain Pose raise the arms above the head, bend the knees, and lower the torso as if sitting down onto a high stool, coming into Chair Pose (*Utkatasana*). Keep the ears between the arms and do not round the upper back. Imagine that your hips are being pulled downward and everything above the waist is reaching skyward. Stay for a few breaths.

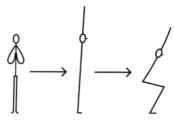

Mountain Pose into Chair Pose

10. *Standing Forward Bend* (Uttanasana)

From Chair Pose (*Utkatasana*) allow your body to melt down into a Standing Forward Bend (*Uttanasana*). Stay here for a few breaths.

Standing Forward Bend

11. *Downward-Facing Dog Pose* (Adho Mukha Svanasana)

From the Standing Forward Bend (*Uttanasana*), walk the hands forward along the mat coming into Downward-Facing Dog Pose (*Adho Mukha Svanasana*). Stay here for a few breaths.

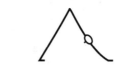

Downward-Facing Dog Pose

12. *Child's Pose* (Balasana) *into Upward-Facing Dog Pose* (Urdhva Mukha Svanasana)

From Downward-Facing Dog Pose (*Adho Mukha Svanasana*), bend the knees, coming onto all fours, and sit back into Child's Pose (*Balasana*), arms outstretched along the floor. Inhale and move forward into Upward-Facing Dog Pose (*Urdhva Mukha Svanasana*), arching your back and keeping your knees on the floor. Exhale back into Child's Pose. You can silently coordinate the breath and movement with the affirmation. Inhale and affirm, *Love surrounds*. Exhale and affirm, *All my feelings*. Repeat 6 times as you move between the two poses. Then rest a few breaths in Child's Pose.

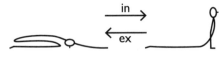

Child's Pose into Upward-Facing Dog Pose

13. *Seated Forward Bend* (Paschimottanasana)

Sit tall, legs outstretched (bend the knees to ease the pose). Inhaling, raise the arms. Exhaling, fold forward over the legs. Inhaling, return to starting position. You can silently coordinate the breath and movement with the affirmation. Inhale and affirm, *Love surrounds*. Exhale and affirm, *All my feelings*. Repeat 6 times, and on the final time stay for a few breaths in the pose. *Finish here or, if you have time, do the Universal Wind-Down Routine in chapter 1.*

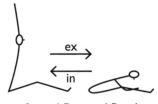

Seated Forward Bend

14. *Short relaxation or Circulation of Light Visualization*

Either go straight to relaxation or do the Circulation of Light Visualization that follows.

Scorpio-Inspired Yoga Practice Overview

1. Mountain Pose.

2. *Ha* breath × 3–6.

3. Push-Away Pose × 6 on each side, alternating sides.

4. Lion Pose × 4.

5. Dynamic Side Bend × 6 on each side.

6. Extended Side Angle Pose.

7. Wood-Chop Squat with *Ha* breathing × 6.

8. Half-Moon Pose.

9. Mountain Pose into Chair Pose.

10. Standing Forward Bend.

11. Downward-Facing Dog Pose.

12. Child's Pose into Upward-Facing Dog Pose × 6.

13. Seated Forward Bend × 6. *You may finish your practice here or do the Universal Wind-Down Routine.*

14. Short relaxation or Circulation of Light Visualization.

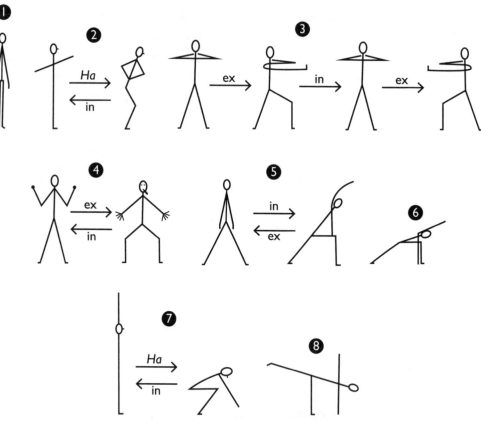

Scorpio-Inspired Yoga Practice Overview

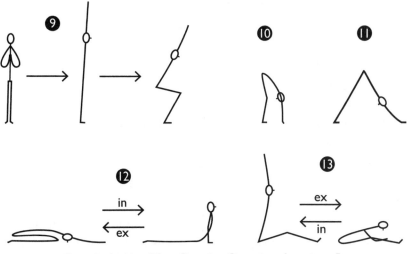

Scorpio-Inspired Yoga Practice Overview (continued)

VISUALIZATION
The Circulation of Light

Scorpio is a sign that pushes us to turn and face life's difficulties. To counterbalance this challenging work, we need to learn the skill of shining light into the darkness, and the Circulation of Light Visualization helps us to do this.

This visualization helps get your energy flowing well through visualizing the circulation of *prana* (subtle energy) around the body. It unblocks stuck, stagnant energy and encourages a healthy, vibrant flow of *prana*, or *chi*. It is energizing and boosts your mood. It also has a stabilizing effect, helping you align and center yourself. In the Northern Hemisphere it is an uplifting way to bring light into the short, dark days of winter.

The visualization can be used on its own, or it's an excellent way to finish your yoga practice, either seated or lying down in Relaxation Pose (*Savasana*). I use it most days to conclude my early morning yoga practice and then follow it with a short *pranayama* practice. Allow 5 to 10 minutes.

Find yourself a comfortable position. If you are sitting, then sit up tall. If you are lying, then check that you are symmetrically arranged around the midline of the spine. You can do this by gently lifting your head and looking along the body; if you notice you're off center, then lower your head and correct the position.

Bring your awareness to the lower belly and imagine a ball of pure white light here. Then visualize that you are circulating this ball of light down around the pelvic floor to the base of the spine, up through the center of the spine to the crown of the head, and then to the space between the brows. Pause briefly here and then take the light energy down the front of the spine and back to the lower belly again. Continue circulating the light in this loop of energy around the body.

If you are new to this visualization, you might prefer to let the breathing take care of itself while you become familiar with the technique of circulating light energy around the body. Once you have gained confidence, you can add a breathing pattern. On the inhale you direct the ball of light from the lower belly around and up the back of the body to between the brows, pausing briefly here, and then exhale, taking the light down the front of the body and back to the lower belly, pausing briefly here. Carry on breathing and visualizing the light circulating in a loop around the front and back of the body. Eventually, it will feel like it is the breath powering the light around the body.

When you feel ready, let go of circulating light around the body and allow your awareness to rest in the lower belly. Notice how the belly rises and falls with each in- and out-breath. Maintain your attention on the rising and falling of the belly and let go of everything else. Allow yourself to breathe and to simply be.

When you are ready, let go of following the breath. Become aware of bodily sensations, particularly noticing the sensations associated with where your body is in contact with the floor or your support. Observe what effect this visualization has had upon you. Do any movements you need to do to wake yourself up. Have a good stretch. When you are ready, carry on with your day.

Scorpio-Inspired Meditation Questions

See chapter 1 for guidance on how to use the meditation questions. The theme for Scorpio is "learning to skillfully ride the waves of change."

- Over the past year what changes have I noticed in myself, those near to me, my surroundings, and the world generally?
    - Imagine what it would be like if nothing ever changed. What would be the downside of everything always remaining the same?
    - What advantageous changes have I noticed recently?

- In what ways does connecting with the natural world help me accept change more willingly?
- When confronted with difficult emotions, what do I find is the best way of managing them?
  - Do I sometimes suppress troublesome emotions, and is that an effective way of dealing with them?
  - Which skills would I need to develop to have the courage to turn and face difficult emotions?
- Which yoga practices give me the stability to live my life courageously and to fight the necessary battles of life?
- When I need to self-soothe, what do I find gives me comfort?
  - Which mindfulness, meditation, or relaxation techniques are helpful?
  - Is there a person who always knows the right thing to say or do to make me feel better?
  - Which activities do I find ground me and help me to feel at ease again?
- What actions would I like to take to connect with others in a loving and supportive way?

CHAPTER 12

The Power of Clear Intention

↗

Sagittarius

November 22–December 21

*Create miracles in your life by narrowing your focus
and connecting to spacious, open, expansive awareness.*

Like an archer drawing back the string of her bow, eye fixed upon the target, yoga teaches us to set our intention. When we practice yoga, we consciously direct our intention to a chosen object. Even though our mind might be flitting all over the place, we continue to draw our attention back to a fixed point, such as the flow of the breath, sensations in the body, or whatever we have chosen to focus on during that session. This concentrated narrowing of our attention leads to an expansive, spacious, state of consciousness.

The experienced archer knows that when she draws the string of her bow, she must always bring it to the same "anchor" point before she releases the arrow, and in this way her shots will be consistent and accurate. Likewise, if our spiritual intention is to hit the target, then consistency and repetition are important anchors. For example, if your

179

intention is to "be kind," each day to enact this you would need to steer your actions toward kindness; you would also need to notice times when you missed opportunities to be kind or acted in an unkind way. Kind acts might include taking time, even though you are very busy, to check in with a colleague at work who's going through a difficult time.

Love, compassion, and kindness are spiritual concepts that can appear rather abstract and airy-fairy. And it's true that if spiritual aspirations aren't backed up by action, they can lapse into sentimentality. Whereas when we set our intention, it brings our spirituality back down to earth and grounds it in lived reality. Small actions performed in a loving way may not be very dramatic, but they all add up to a life well lived. In contrast a generalized ambition, such as a desire to "show love to all humanity," is like an archer shooting an arrow up into the sky, and just crossing his fingers and hoping that it will land on the chosen target.

Intention is a powerful force that can work miracles when combined with wisdom. William Hutchison Murray wrote, "The moment one definitely commits oneself, then Providence moves too. All sorts of things occur to help one that would never otherwise have occurred. A whole stream of events issues from the decision, raising in one's favor all manner of unforeseen incidents and meetings and material assistance, which no man could have dreamt would have come his way."[46]

Yoga expands your vison of what is physically, mentally, and spiritually possible. On a physical level, yoga takes your body to places you never believed possible. For example, in an inverted pose such as Downward-Facing Dog Pose, you look at the world from a different angle, and this upside-down world gives you a fresh perspective. The meditative practices of yoga also turn your world upside-down and challenge your habitual way of viewing the world. In meditation you are connected to nature, the earth, the sky, and the cosmos.

Yoga is as wide as the world and as deep as the ocean. It connects you to a spacious, open, and expansive awareness—something so much bigger than yourself. Paradoxically, to expand your horizon yoga requires that you narrow your focus and sharpen your intention. Before commencing any journey, first we decide on a direction of travel. If we are clear about where we wish to get to, we will be able to correct if we veer off course. New paths open and stretch out to the horizon.

---

46. William Hutchison Murray, *The Scottish Himalayan Expedition* (London: J. M. Dent & Sons, 1951), 6–7.

Yoga Inspired by Sagittarius

Sagittarius is a mutable, positive fire sign, ruled by Jupiter. Its symbol is the centaur with bow and arrow. In India the constellation of Sagittarius was known as Dhanus. In Rome it was associated with Diana, the goddess of the bow.[47] Sagittarian colors are purple and deep blue. Key words are *widely*, *deeply*, and *free-ranging*.

With the rulership of Jupiter, we move away from the fierce life/death intensity of the previous sign, Scorpio, and toward a more jovial, happy-go-lucky outlook. The Breathe and Smile Meditation, to be found later in this chapter, aims to reflect and incorporate the cheerful optimism of this sign. The key words for Jupiter are *expansion* and *preservation*. The god Jupiter was the Roman Heavenly Father, from Sanskrit, *Dyaus pitar*. Juno was Jupiter's wife, and it was thought that every Roman woman embodied a bit of the goddess's spirit in her soul, which was her own unique genius.[48]

The power of the hips and thighs are said to be Sagittarian, and this correlates with the desire to travel far and wide. The sign conjures up images of freedom, wide open spaces, blue skies, and wild horses roaming free across moorland.

The symbol for the sign is a centaur, which is half horse and half human. And this image of half-horse and half-human being can be a powerful one to hold in your mind during a yoga practice, allowing it to inspire your choice of asanas and the quality of your movement. Hindus, Arabs, and Celts considered the horseshoe lucky because of its yonic shape, which they regarded as a symbol of the Goddess's "Great Gate." Some Hindu temples were constructed in the shape of a horseshoe with the frank intention of representing the *yoni*. The yonic horseshoe shape can also be related to the last letter of the Greek sacred alphabet, omega, or "Great Om," the Word of Creation beginning the next cycle of creation. The implication of the horseshoe symbol was that having entered the yonic door at the end of life (omega), man would be reborn as a new child (alpha) through the same door.[49] Even today a horseshoe on a door is considered to be lucky, although those who reside within are unlikely to realize the origin of the symbol and its feminine connotations.

MacNeice writes that the fire of Sagittarius is the purifying blue fire at the heart of the flame, and this can be a beautiful image to explore and seek out in art and poetry.[50]

---

47. Walker, *The Woman's Dictionary of Symbols and Sacred Objects*, 293.

48. Walker, *The Woman's Encyclopedia of Myths and Secrets*, 484–85.

49. Walker, *The Woman's Encyclopedia of Myths and Secrets*, 414–15.

50. MacNeice, *Astrology*, 96.

In the Northern Hemisphere the Sagittarian dates correspond with our entering into the depths of winter, so this blue flame image, when introduced into a yoga practice or meditation, can be a way of bringing light into the darkness.

It can be enriching for the yoga practitioner to find out more about the skills and discipline of archery, some of which are very similar to those we cultivate in yoga, such as balancing effort (*sthira*) and relaxation (*sukha*).

Sagittarius-Inspired Yoga Practice

In the Sagittarius-inspired yoga practice that follows I have chosen asanas inspired by archery imagery. We combine the arm movements of drawing your bow and releasing an arrow with familiar poses such as the Lunge Pose (*Anjaneyasana*) and Warrior Pose (*Virabhadrasana*). We also explore the tautness of the archer's bow through poses such as a Lunge Pose variation and Bow Pose (*Dhanurasana*). The practice is calming, grounding, centering, and energizing and improves focus.

The affirmation we use in the practice is *My intention is clear, and opportunities arise.* It can be coordinated with the breath:

Inhale: Clear intention

Exhale: Opportunities arise

Allow 20 to 30 minutes.

1. Mountain Pose (Tadasana)

Stand tall, feet parallel and about hip width apart. Be aware of the contact between your feet and the earth beneath you. Imagine a string attached to the crown of your head, gently pulling you skyward; simultaneously, let your tailbone drop and feel your heels rooting down into the earth. Be aware of the space around you. Silently repeat the affirmation 3 times: *My intention is clear, and opportunities arise.*

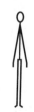

Mountain Pose

If you feel the need to warm up to prepare for the practice, then use the Universal Warm-Up Routine in chapter 1.

2. *Warrior 1* (**Virabhadrasana 1**)

Stand tall, feet hip width apart. Turn your right foot out slightly and take a big step forward with your left foot. Inhaling, raise both arms above your head and bend the left knee over the ankle. Exhaling, lower the arms and straighten the leg. Do 6 repetitions on this side, and on the final time stay for a few breaths with the arms raised. Then repeat on the other side. You can coordinate the breath with the affirmation. Inhale and affirm, *Clear intention.* Exhale and affirm, *Opportunities arise.*

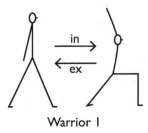

Warrior I

3. *Dancer Pose* (**Natarajasana**) *variation*

Stand tall, feet hip width apart and arms by your sides. Bend your right knee, and with your right hand catch hold of your ankle. Either take the left arm out to the side at shoulder height or up above the head. Stay for a few breaths and then repeat on the other side. (This modified variation of the Dancer Pose [*Natarajasana*] is slightly easier than the full version in step 5 when we tip the torso forward into a back bend.)

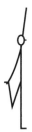

Dancer Pose variation

4. *Warrior Archer Pose* (Virabhadrasana *variation*)

Stand tall, feet hip width apart. Turn your right foot out slightly and take a big step forward with your left foot. Raise both arms forward to shoulder level and bring the fingertips together. Inhaling, bend the right arm, draw an imaginary bow, and straighten the arm behind you, palm facing out. Exhale and close the straight right arm back to the starting position. Repeat 6 times. Then repeat on the other side.

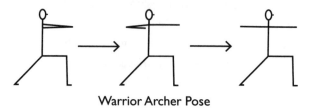

Warrior Archer Pose

5. *Dancer Pose* (Natarajasana)

Come into Dancer Pose variation (see step 3). From here tip the torso forward, extending the back foot up and away from you and reaching forward and up with the opposite arm. Stay for a few breaths and then repeat on the other side. If you have balance problems, practice facing a wall, with your extended hand resting on the wall for support.

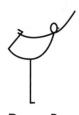

Dancer Pose

6. *Chair Pose* (Utkatasana)

Stand tall, feet hip width apart and both arms above your head. Bend your knees and lower your bottom as if to sit down on a high stool. Keep the ears between the arms and do not round the upper back. Imagine that your hips are being pulled downward and everything above the waist is reaching skyward. Stay for a few breaths.

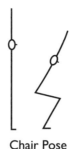

Chair Pose

7. Lunge Archer Pose (Anjaneyasana *variation*)

Come to tall kneeling. Take your left foot forward, bend the knee, and bring the knee over the ankle. Raise both arms forward to shoulder level and bring the fingertips together. Inhaling, bend the right arm, draw an imaginary bow, and straighten the arm behind you, palm facing out. Exhaling, close the straight right arm back to the starting position. Repeat 6 times. Then repeat on the other side.

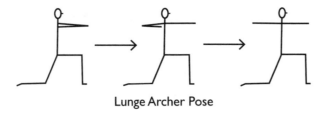

Lunge Archer Pose

8. Puppy Dog Pose (Uttana Shishosana) *into Child's Pose* (Balasana)

Come onto all fours. Walk the hands forward along the floor, until your arms, head, and torso form one long diagonal line, keeping the thighs at a 90-degree angle. Keep the ears between the arms. Stay here for a few breaths. Then bend the knees, sit the bottom back onto the heels, and rest for a few breaths in Child's Pose (*Balasana*).

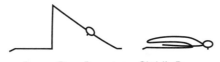

Puppy Dog Pose into Child's Pose

9a. *Lunge Pose* (Anjaneyasana)

Come to tall kneeling. Take your right foot forward, bending the right knee over the ankle. Either take your hands to the heart in the Prayer Position (Namaste) or raise the arms above the head. Stay here for a few breaths. Repeat on the other side.

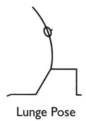

Lunge Pose

9b. *Lunge Pose holding ankle* (Anjaneyasana *variation*)

Come into the Lunge Pose with your right foot forward. Bend your left leg and bring the heel toward the buttock. Take both hands behind you to catch hold of the ankle. Stay here for a few breaths. Repeat on the other side.

If you have any knee problems, skip 9b and go straight to 10.

Lunge Pose holding ankle

10. *Downward-Facing Dog* (Adho Mukha Svanasana)

From the Lunge Pose, place both hands on the floor on either side of the front foot, turn the toes of the back foot under, and step the front foot back into Downward-Facing Dog. Stay here for a few breaths.

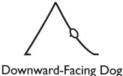

Downward-Facing Dog

11. *Bow Pose* (Dhanurasana) *variation*

Lie on your front, arms by your sides. Inhale, lifting your chest and bending both knees. Exhale, lowering your chest and straightening legs back to the floor. Repeat 6 times and stay in the final pose for a few breaths.

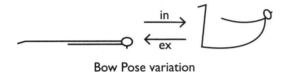

Bow Pose variation

12. *Bow Pose* (Dhanurasana)

Lie on your front, arms by your sides. Bend both knees and catch hold of your ankles. Lift your chest and knees up and away from the floor, gently pulling your shoulders back to open the chest. If comfortable, stay here for a few breaths. Then lower down to the floor, release the ankles, straighten your legs along the floor, and turn your head to one side, resting for a few breaths.

If you wish to work at a gentler level, then skip step 12 or repeat step 11.

Bow Pose

13. *Cat Pose* (Marjaryasana) *into Child's Pose* (Balasana)

Come onto all fours. Exhaling, round the back into Cat Pose (*Marjaryasana*) and lower the bottom to the heels and the head to the floor into Child's Pose (*Balasana*). Inhaling, come back up to all fours. Repeat 6 times. You can coordinate the breath with the affirmation. Inhale and affirm, *Clear intention.* Exhale and affirm, *Opportunities arise.*

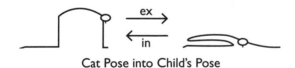

Cat Pose into Child's Pose

14. *Child's Pose* (Balasana)

Rest for a few breaths here. *Finish here or move on to step 15.*

Child's Pose

15. *Universal Wind-Down Routine and Breathe and Smile Meditation*

Conclude with the Universal Wind-Down Routine in chapter 1. And if you have time, do the Breathe and Smile Meditation (see page 190).

Sagittarius-Inspired Yoga Practice Overview

1. Mountain Pose with affirmation: *My intention is clear, and opportunities arise.*
2. Warrior 1 × 6 on this side. On final time stay a few breaths. Repeat on other side. Inhale: *Clear intention.* Exhale: *Opportunities arise.*
3. Dancer Pose variation. Stay a few breaths. Repeat on other side.
4. Warrior Archer Pose × 6. Repeat on other side.
5. Dancer Pose.
6. Chair Pose.
7. Lunge Archer Pose × 6. Repeat on other side.
8. Puppy Dog Pose. Stay a few breaths. Child's Pose. Rest a few breaths.
9a. Lunge Pose.
9b. Lunge Pose holding ankle. *Skip step for a gentler practice.*
10. Downward-Facing Dog. Stay a few breaths.
11. Bow Pose variation × 6. Stay in final pose for a few breaths.
12. Bow Pose. Stay for a few breaths. *Skip step for a gentler practice.*
13. Cat Pose into Child's Pose × 6. Inhale: *Clear intention.* Exhale: *Opportunities arise.*
14. Child's Pose. Rest a few breaths. *Finish here or move on to step 15.*
15. Universal Wind-Down and Breathe and Smile Meditation.

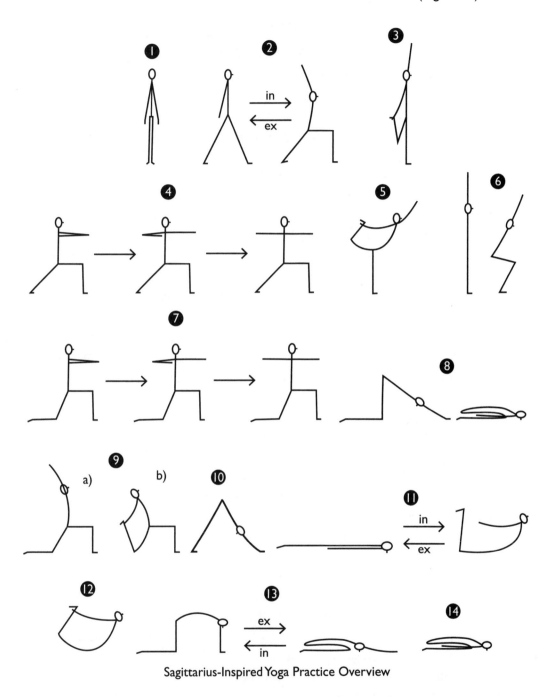

Sagittarius-Inspired Yoga Practice Overview

MEDITATION
Breathe and Smile

Sometimes we approach our meditation practice with such intensity that we forget to cultivate an attitude of joyfulness. The Breathe and Smile Meditation allows you to maintain a clear, focused attention while at the same time joyfully lightening up. The meditation fits in with the cheerful optimism and joviality that is associated with Sagittarius.

This meditation can be done sitting on the floor or in a chair or lying in Relaxation Pose (*Savasana*). Allow 10 minutes.

Find yourself a comfortable position, either sitting or lying down. Become aware of your body, particularly noticing which parts are in contact with the floor or your support. If you notice any discomfort in your body, be aware of it without immediately trying to fix it. Notice any sensations associated with the discomfort and how they change from breath to breath. Notice which parts of your body already feel relaxed, comfortable, and at ease.

Become aware of the natural flow of the breath. Notice where in your body you are most aware of the movement of the breath. Perhaps you feel it at the nostrils as the air enters and leaves the body, or perhaps you can sense it in the chest or the belly. Wherever you feel it most clearly, allow your awareness to settle there for a few breaths.

Next picture someone or something that makes you smile. Perhaps it is one of your kids, a grandchild, a pet, or a best friend. Allow your lips to relax into a smile; notice how a smile relaxes so many of the facial muscles. Imagine that the smile is spreading through your body: your eyes are smiling; the back of your throat is smiling; the smile expands across your chest; your belly is smiling. If any part of your body needs soothing, imagine that part of your body is relaxing into a smile.

Return your awareness again to the natural flow of your breath. Particularly, be aware of the out-breath, which is the part of the breath associated with relaxation. Each time you breathe out, feel yourself relaxing into a half smile. A half smile is that gentle smile that you see on the face of the Buddha. So, you take a breath in, and on each exhale you smile. Continue over a few more breaths with that rhythm of inhaling, exhaling, smiling.

Now imagine that the air you breathe comes from a vast ocean of love. With each inhale you draw love into yourself, and with each exhale give love back to the world. Inhale: *Love*. Exhale: *Love*. Carry on for a few more breaths and then let it go.

Notice what effect this meditation has had upon you. In what way do you feel different now than how you felt at the start of the meditation?

To conclude become aware of your body, noticing any sensations associated with the contact between your body and the floor or your support. Feel a connection to the earth beneath you. Become aware of your surroundings. Do any movements you need to do to wake yourself up, including a good stretch. Resolve to stay in touch with your inner smile as you go about your day.

Sagittarius-Inspired Meditation Questions

See chapter 1 for guidance on how to use the meditation questions. The theme is "developing focus and concentration and setting your intention."

- What are the advantages and disadvantages of making a commitment (to work, relationships, study, a hobby, yoga, etc.)?
  - What are the advantages and disadvantages of flitting from one thing to another?
- Are there any areas of my life that would benefit from me having a clear intention of the direction I want to follow?
- What are the differences between setting my intention and having a fixed goal in mind?
- How can I best place myself to take full advantage of opportunities that arise and so fulfill my potential?
- What lights my fire, and what am I passionate about?
  - How can I best steer myself in the direction of following my passions?
- What do I most value in my relationships?
  - What gets in the way of me living by these values?
  - What small steps could I take to move a relationship in a positive direction?
- What are my aims in practicing yoga?
  - Choosing one of these aims, how would I phrase it as a simple intention to use to guide a yoga session?
- Which yoga techniques help improve my focus and concentration?

CHAPTER 13

Transcend Limitations
and Find Liberation

♑
Capricorn
December 21–January 20
Discover the opportunities hidden within your difficulties,
and open the door to self-discovery.

Yoga brings us face to face with our limitations and opens the door to exploring fresh ways of working with these restrictions. Our willingness to acknowledge our limitations opens new possibilities of freedom and liberation. We find that in the middle of difficulty lies opportunity.

Sometimes in life it can feel as though every door has been shut in our face. We feel heavy, despondent, and lost. Yoga teaches us to rest in the pause. We learn to trust that like the New Moon appearing in the night sky, new life will emerge from the darkness.

Yoga is there at those times when life feels like a blank page and no words come. The ink has dried up, and you fear inspiration has run dry. At times when you are filled with self-doubt and feel all used up, yoga is there like the Sun appearing on the horizon at the start of a new day.

The way we approach a challenging yoga pose often mirrors how we deal with life's challenges generally. In a difficult yoga pose we come face to face with our habitual way of reacting to struggle; this opens the door to exiting a negative cycle of reaction and finding a new way of responding.

In asana practice we are continually exploring our boundaries. We discover how far we can push in a pose before we come up against our physical limitations. Then we must decide whether to push further to the point of pain or to back off and come back to our edge. The edge is the place where you feel a stretch, perhaps even mild discomfort, but you haven't jumped off the cliff edge into pain.

For some people a yoga asana becomes an enemy to be conquered. Pain is regarded as weakness and something to be pushed through to gain victory over the pose. However, if your experience of a pose is all push and no yield, then you miss out on the peace of yoga. Likewise, in life when challenges come up, if you react by telling yourself "get a grip" or "man up," you miss out on the warmth of human connection that comes from revealing your softer, more vulnerable side.

Yoga teaches us how to discover the opportunities that lie dormant within our difficulties. When you attempt a challenging yoga pose, you are confronted with your physical, mental, and emotional limitations. If you listen, each asana will teach you how to respond rather than react to whatever arises. Then the skills we learn on the mat can be transferred to responding more skillfully when difficulties arise in life. In this way yoga can be a doorway to self-discovery.

In the silent stillness of meditation, a door opens, leading into the subconscious and universal conscious. In this deeply relaxed, awakened yogic state we gain access to the body's subtle energy centers (chakras) which in turn are a doorway to the soul.

- The root chakra (*muladhara*) is the door to the ancestors and the instinctual self.
- The creation chakra (*svadhisthana*) is the door to gut feelings, intuition, and the flow of creation.
- The solar plexus chakra (*manipura*) is the door to personal power, integrity, and self-worth.
- The heart chakra (*anahata*) is the door to love and relationships.
- The throat chakra (*vishuddha*) is the door to communication and the mantra *Om*.

- The third eye chakra (*ajna*) is the door to intuition, knowing, and clear sight.

- The crown chakra (*sahasrara*) is the doorway to bliss and enlightenment.

Yoga Inspired by Capricorn

Capricorn is a cardinal earth sign, ruled by Saturn. Its symbol is a mythical sea-goat. Its metal is lead, and its colors are black and dark hues. The parts of the body assigned to it are the skeletal system and the skin, and the time of life is old age. Its key words are *prudently, coolly,* and *aspiringly.*

The Capricorn symbol is a goat with a fish tail, which in Sanskrit was *Makara,* the sea monster.[51] The lower half is a fish which can plumb the depths of the sea, and we can relate to the depths of the subconscious mind. Its upper half is a goat, which can nimbly scale mountain peaks and takes us from the inner world of the mind back out into the outside world.

The sign has an association with gates and doors. A door can lead us inside to an interior world; we can also pass through it to go out into the world. In India doorways and entrances are often demarked with women's ritual drawings called *kolam*—ground rice flower designs in white—which mark space and thresholds. These beautiful women's ritual designs also mark time: dawn and dusk and the month of the winter solstice.[52] Capricorn teaches us that as one door closes, another door opens.

In the Northern Hemisphere Capricorn dates correspond with the winter solstice, and the darkness and coldness of this season may explain the sign's association with old age. The winter landscape can be bleak, everything has died back, and it's icy cold. In yoga terms this is the heavy energy of *tamas* (the black thread of creation) and the Crone aspect of the birth-life-death-rebirth cycle. In our yoga practice we can work with this heaviness by contrasting it with lightness and images of light.

During the period of Capricorn, we leave behind the old year and walk through the doorway into a new year. The period between the ending of the old year and the beginning of the new one is an in-between time, a pause. Capricorn teaches us to learn to rest in that empty space between an ending and a new beginning. The pause can be a scary, bewildering place, especially if your default mode is keeping busy. The wisdom of Capricorn is that if you can allow yourself to fully experience emptiness, you create a space for

---

51. Walker, *The Woman's Dictionary of Symbols and Sacred Objects,* 290.

52. Tracy Pintchman, *Women's Lives, Women's Rituals in the Hindu Tradition* (New York: Oxford University Press, 2007), 86.

new life, and new energy, to fill you up. It's the medicine you need when you feel all used up, all energy spent, nothing more to give. If you can relax into this emptiness, if you can trust the pause, you will find that new ideas and fresh inspiration will come to fill you up again. The peace of the pause opens the door to rejuvenation and renewal.

Capricorn can be compared to the pause between the out-breath and the next in-breath. In yoga breathing, this pause between the breaths is the place where we find peace, rest, and renewal. It is the place where we allow our self to be emptied, creating the space for new life, new energy, to fill us up. We are literally inspired.

In his book *Astrology*, Louis MacNeice refers to Capricorn as "the gate to spiritual life," as "under Capricorn, like a yogi, one practices control," and he considered that with this sign we "are on the brink of spiritual rebirth."[53] Saturn's rulership imposes boundaries and limitations, and it is the overcoming of these obstacles that gives us the opportunity for spiritual growth and opens the door to freedom.

Capricorn-Inspired Yoga Practice

In the Capricorn-inspired yoga practice that follows I have included asanas that restrict and bind the body, such as Eagle Pose (*Garudasana*) and Cow Face Pose (*Gomukhasana*). These restrictive poses give us the opportunity to relax into difficulty and so find the freedom inherent within the pose. This is contrasted with opening, expansive poses, which echo the Capricorn theme of doors opening and closing and the idea of working with our limitations and rising above them. This in turn opens the door to transformation, and life comes alive again.

The affirmation we use in the practice is *I am open to new possibilities.* It can be coordinated with the breath:

Inhale: I am open

Exhale: To new possibilities

Allow 20 to 30 minutes.

1. Mountain Pose (Tadasana)

Stand tall, feet parallel and about hip width apart. Be aware of the contact between your feet and the earth beneath you. Imagine a string attached to the crown of your head, gen-

---

53. MacNeice, *Astrology*, 100.

tly pulling you skyward; simultaneously, let your tailbone drop and feel your heels rooting down into the earth. Silently repeat this affirmation: *I am open to new possibilities.*

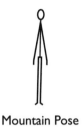

Mountain Pose

2. Capricorn Opening and Closing Doors Sequence

Follow these steps for the Capricorn Opening and Closing Doors Sequence:

2a. Bend and straighten warm-up

Take the legs 2 to 3 feet apart and turn the toes slightly out. Take the arms out to the sides at shoulder height, palms facing downward. On your next exhale, bend the knees and lower the arms. Inhale, returning to the starting position. You can silently coordinate the breath and movement with the affirmation. Inhale: *I am open.* Exhale: *To new possibilities.* Repeat 6 times.

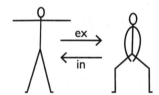

Bend and straighten warm-up

2b. Dynamic Side Bend

With the legs 2 to 3 feet apart and arms by your sides, turn the toes slightly out. Inhale as you bend your left knee, and raise your right arm overhead, side-bending to the right. Exhale, lower the arm, straighten the leg, returning to the starting position. Repeat 6 times. On the final time stay for a few breaths in the side bend.

Before you go on to the other side, do 2c (Eagle Pose Arms, right arm on top), 2d (Cow Face Pose Arms, right arm on top), and 2e (Opening and Closing Doors Pose).

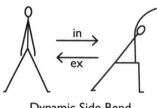

Dynamic Side Bend

2c. Eagle Pose Arms (Garudasana *variation*)

From the side bend, come into Eagle Pose Arms by extending both arms out in front, parallel to the floor. Place the right arm over the left, bend the elbows, nestling the right elbow into the crook of the left, and bring the backs of the hands together or clasp the palms together. Gently raise the elbows a little, keeping the shoulders down and creating length in the back of the neck. Keeping the Eagle Pose Arms, exhale and bend the knees, and inhale into starting position. Repeat 4 times.

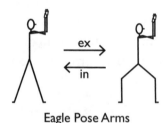

Eagle Pose Arms

2d. Cow Face Pose Arms (Gomukhasana *variation*)

From Eagle Pose Arms, stretch the right arm up toward the ceiling, then bend the arm, placing the right hand at the top of the spine, fingers pointing downward and palm turned in. Take your left arm behind your back, palm turned outward, and ease the lower left hand up along the length of the spine toward the top hand, as you ease the right hand down toward the left. If you are very flexible, you may be able to hook the fingers together. Hold the pose, stretching the right elbow up toward the ceiling and descending the left elbow down toward the floor. Stay here for a few breaths and then release the arms.

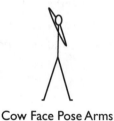

Cow Face Pose Arms

2e. Opening and Closing Doors Pose

From Cow Face Pose Arms (*Gomukhasana* variation), take the arms out to the sides at shoulder height and bend them, forming a right angle at the elbow, fingers pointing up toward the ceiling and palms facing forward. Exhale, bend the knees, and bring the fore-arms and hands together in front of the chest (doors closed). Inhale, straighten the legs, and "open the doors" by bringing the arms back to the starting position. Repeat 6 times.

Repeat 2b through 2e, moving the left arm this time.

If you are pushed for time, finish your practice here.

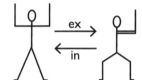

Opening and Closing Doors Pose

3. Eagle Pose (Garudasana)

Stand in Mountain Pose (*Tadasana*). Bend your knees, lift your left foot up, cross your left thigh over your right, and, if you can, hook the top of the left foot behind the lower right calf. Extend both arms out in front, parallel to the floor. Place the right arm over the left, bend the elbows, nestling the right elbow into the crook of the left, and bring the backs of the hands together or clasp the palms together. Gently raise the elbows a little, keeping the shoulders down and creating length in the back of the neck. Stay for a few breaths. Repeat on the other side.

Eagle Pose

4. Standing Twist (Parivrtta Trikonasana) Combination Sequence

Take the legs 2 to 3 feet apart, feet parallel and arms out to the side and parallel to the floor. Exhale and come into a Standing Twist (*Parivrtta Trikonasana*) by bending for-ward from the hip joints, taking one hand to the floor (or to the leg for gentler pose), and raising the other arm up toward the ceiling. Look up at the raised hand. Stay here for one breath, lengthening through the spine as you twist. Inhale and come back up to standing, arms out to the side. Repeat on the other side. Inhale and come back up to standing, arms out to the side. Exhale and bend forward from the hip joint into Wide-Leg Standing Forward Bend Pose (*Prasarita Padottanasana*), bringing the hands to the floor (for a gentler version bring the hands to rest on the legs). Inhale and come back up to standing, arms out to the sides. Repeat the entire Standing Twist Combination Sequence 3 more times.

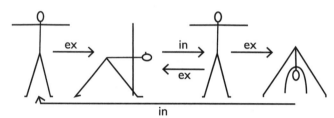

Standing Twist Combination Sequence

5. Cow Face Pose (Gomukhasana)

Sit with your legs stretched out in front of you, then bend your knees, keeping the soles of the feet on floor. Tuck your left foot under the right knee, bringing it to the outside of the right buttock, and cross your right leg over the left, bringing the right foot onto the outside of the left hip, right knee pointing up toward the ceiling. Sit evenly balanced on both sitting bones.

Take your right arm behind your back, bending the arm and bringing the back of the hand to rest on the lower spine. Slide the hand up the back until it is between the shoulder blades, or below. Keep the right elbow in toward the right side of your torso. Stretch your left arm straight up toward the ceiling, palm turned back, then bend the elbow and reach down the spine for the right hand. If possible, hook the right and left fingers. Lift the left elbow up toward the ceiling and descend the right elbow down toward the floor. Stay in the pose for a few breaths, silently repeating this affirmation: *I am open to new possibilities*. Repeat on the other side.

Cow Face Pose

6. *Seated Forward Bend* (**Paschimottanasana**)

Sit tall, legs outstretched (bend the knees to ease the pose). Inhaling, raise both arms. Exhaling, fold forward over the legs. Inhaling, return to starting position. You can silently coordinate the breath and movement with the affirmation. Inhale and affirm, *I am open*. Exhale and affirm, *To new possibilities*. Repeat 6 times, and on the final time stay for a few breaths in the pose.

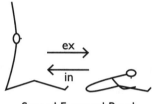

Seated Forward Bend

7. *Half-Locust Pose* (**Ardha Salabhasana**)

Lie on your front, with your head facing down and arms by your sides. Inhale to prepare. Exhale and raise the upper body into a backbend, sweeping the arms out to the side like a bird's wings; at the same time lift one straight leg from the floor (keep both frontal pelvic bones on the floor—do not twist the pelvis as you come into the backbend). Inhale and lift the chest a little higher. Exhale and lower to the starting position. Repeat on the other side. Repeat 4 times on each side, alternating sides.

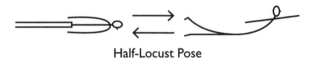

Half-Locust Pose

8. *Sphinx Pose* (**Salamba Bhujangasana**)

Lying on your front, come up into a gentle backbend, propping yourself up on your forearms. Remember not to crease the back of the neck. Feel the tailbone and the crown of the head lengthening away from each other. Be aware of the natural rhythm of the breath. Stay here for a few breaths, silently repeating the affirmation: *I am open to new possibilities*.

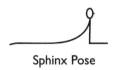

Sphinx Pose

9. *Child's Pose* (Balasana)

Rest for a few breaths here. Be particularly aware of the exhale, noticing the pause between each exhale and the next inhale. With each exhale feel yourself relaxing a little more deeply.

Finish here or move on to step 10.

Child's Pose

10. *Universal Wind-Down Routine and meditation*

Conclude with the Universal Wind-Down Routine in chapter 1. If you have time, you could do either the Door to Freedom Chakra Meditation that follows or another meditation or relaxation of your choice.

Capricorn-Inspired Yoga Practice Overview

1. Mountain Pose with affirmation: *I am open to new possibilities.*
2. Capricorn Opening and Closing Doors Sequence:

    2a. Bend and straighten warm-up × 6. Inhale: *I am open.* Exhale: *To new possibilities.*

    2b. Dynamic Side Bend × 6. On final time stay a few breaths.

    2c. Eagle Pose Arms × 4, right arm on top.

    2d. Cow Face Pose Arms, right arm on top.

    2e. Opening and Closing Doors × 6.

    Repeat 2b through 2e, moving the left arm this time. If pushed for time, finish here.
3. Eagle Pose. Stay for a few breaths. Repeat on other side.
4. Standing Twist Combination sequence × 4.
5. Cow Face Pose with affirmation: *I am open to new possibilities.*
6. Seated Forward Bend. Inhale: *I am open.* Exhale: *To new possibilities.* Repeat × 6.
7. Half-Locust Pose × 4 on each side, alternating sides.
8. Sphinx Pose. Stay for a few breaths, with affirmation: *I am open to new possibilities.*
9. Child's Pose. Rest here for a few breaths. *Finish here or move on to step 10.*

10. Universal Wind-Down Routine. If time, Door to Freedom Chakra Meditation or another meditation or relaxation of your choice.

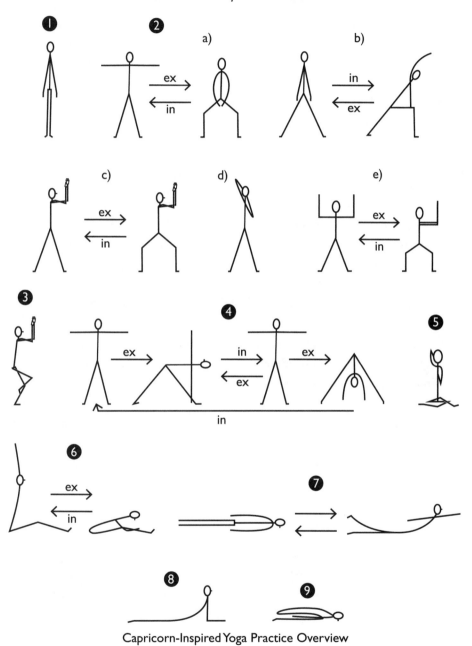

Capricorn-Inspired Yoga Practice Overview

MEDITATION

MEDITATION
Door to Freedom Chakra Meditation

Capricorn is associated with gates and doors, which is why I have chosen this Door to Freedom Chakra Meditation, with its theme of opening the door to enlightenment. The chakras are poetically described as lotus flowers connected by their stems to the *Sushumna,* which is the subtle energy channel to be found within the spinal column. Meditating upon the chakras opens a door to a heightened awareness of the interconnection between the material and more subtle layers of existence. In this meditation we use color and sound to step through the door that connects the material, mental, emotional, and spiritual sides of our being.

This meditation encourages a healthy, unblocked flow of energy; enhances the blossoming of creativity; energizes and uplifts; and has a balancing effect, bringing you back in alignment, both physically, mentally, and spiritually. It creates the right conditions for the door to enlightenment to open.

Allow 15 to 20 minutes for this meditation.

Each chakra has a *bija* (meaning "seed") mantra associated with it, used for meditation. The beauty of these simple seed mantras is that they are accessible, and it doesn't matter whether you can sing in tune or not. It's worth noting that the final *M* sound in all the seed mantras is prolonged, like a humming sound.

Find yourself a comfortable sitting position, either cross-legged on the floor or on a straight-backed chair. Ground yourself by becoming aware of where your body is in contact with the floor or your support; relax into the support of the earth beneath you. Sit up tall. Feel the spine lengthening. Be aware of the centerline of the body and arrange yourself symmetrically around this midline.

The meditation is done in seven stages, taking us up the seven chakras, from root to crown. This is then reversed, and we finish the meditation by traveling down the seven chakras from crown back to root.

1. Root Chakra (*Muladhara*): Rest your awareness in the area between the base of the spine and the pubic bone. Picture a red flower here in full bloom. Inhale, and on the exhale chant *Lam* (pronounced *lum*). Repeat the chant twice more.

2. Creation Chakra (*Svadhisthana*): Rest your awareness in the lower belly, the area between the pubic bone and the navel. Picture an orange flower here in full bloom. Inhale, and on the exhale chant *Vam* (pronounced *vum*). Repeat the chant twice more.

3. Solar Plexus Chakra (*Manipura*): Rest your awareness in the solar plexus, the area above the navel but below the breastbone. Picture a yellow flower here in full bloom. Inhale, and on the exhale chant *Ram* (pronounced *rum*). Repeat the chant twice more.

4. Heart Center Chakra (*Anahata*): Rest your awareness at the heart center. Picture a pink lotus flower on a bed of green leaves here. Inhale, and on the exhale chant *Yam* (pronounced *yum*). Repeat the chant twice more.

5. Communication Chakra (*Vishuddha*): Bring your awareness to the throat. Picture a blue flower here in full bloom. Inhale, and on the exhale chant *Ham* (pronounced *hum*). Repeat the chant twice more.

6. Third Eye Chakra (*Ajna*): Bring your awareness to the area between the brows. Picture a purple flower here in full bloom. Inhale, and on the exhale chant *Am* (pronounced *um*). Repeat the chant twice more.

7. Crown Chakra (*Sahasrara*): Bring your awareness to the area just above the crown of the head. Picture a pure white lotus flower here in full bloom. Inhale, and on the exhale chant *Om* (pronounced *aum*). Repeat the chant twice more.

Stay here, your awareness resting with all the seven chakras, and simultaneously maintaining a gentle, background awareness of the natural flow of the breath.

To conclude the meditation, we travel back down through the chakras from the crown to the root chakra, at each chakra silently chanting the seed mantras and closing the chakra flower back to bud.

1. Crown Chakra (*Sahasrara*): Inhale, on the exhale silently chant *Om* (pronounced *aum*). Repeat twice more. Picture a white lotus flower closing back to bud.

2. Third Eye Chakra (*Ajna*): Inhale, on the exhale silently chant *Am* (pronounced *um*). Repeat twice more. Picture a purple flower closing back to bud.

3. Communication Chakra (*Vishuddha*): Inhale, on the exhale silently chant *Ham* (pronounced *hum*). Repeat twice more. Picture a blue flower here closing back to bud.

4. Heart Chakra (*Anahata*): Inhale, on the exhale silently chant *Yam* (pronounced *yum*). Repeat twice more. Picture a pink lotus flower on a bed of green leaves here closing back to bud.

5. Solar Plexus Chakra (*Manipura*): Inhale, on the exhale silently chant *Ram* (pronounced *rum*). Repeat the chant twice more. Picture a yellow flower here closing back to bud.

6. Creation Chakra (*Svadisthana*): Inhale, on the exhale silently chant *Vam* (pronounced *vum*). Repeat the chant twice more. Picture an orange flower here closing back to bud.

7. Root Chakra (*Muladhara*): Inhale, on the exhale silently chant *Lam* (pronounced *lum*). Repeat the chant twice more. Picture a red flower here closing back to bud.

Sit quietly for a few more breaths, noticing how the meditation has affected you. Then bring your thumbs and index fingers together to create a downward-pointing triangle (*Yoni Mudra*). Rest the *Yoni Mudra* hands on the lower belly. Stay here for a few breaths. Then form the hands into a lotus shape, little fingers and thumbs touching, other fingers spread wide like open petals (this is *Padma Mudra*). Hold the lotus shape hands at the heart center. Then curl the fingers together like a flower closing back to bud. Stay here for a few more breaths. Rest the hands back in the lap. When you are ready, have a good stretch and carry on with your day.

Capricorn-Inspired Meditation Questions

See chapter 1 for guidance on how to use the meditation questions. The theme is "opening doors and overcoming limitations."

• What doors has my yoga practice opened for me?
• What is my response when confronted with a challenging yoga pose?
  – How does this mirror the way I respond or react to difficulties in life?

- Are there any yoga poses (or aspects of yoga) that I believe are impossible for me?
  - Would visualizing myself in this challenging pose help make it seem more possible for me?
  - Even if I cannot achieve a pose, are there small preparatory steps I could take toward achieving it?
- When I am feeling heavy, despondent, and burdened, how might yoga lighten my mood?
  - What other ways have I found of making life come alive again?
- What are the limitations that I face in life?
  - Would visualizing myself overcoming these limitations help inspire me with ideas for overcoming the difficulty?
  - What small steps could I take toward changing the situation and removing the obstacle?
- How comfortable am I with setting boundaries?
  - In what ways would setting boundaries make my life easier and more enjoyable?
- Have there been times in my life when facing a difficulty has revealed hidden opportunities and led to a new beginning?

CHAPTER 14

Drawing from the Wellspring of Love

Aquarius

January 20–February 19

Combine science, creativity, and love to bring healing to yourself and the world.

Yoga is like a waterfall that flows into a river: generous and non-judgmental, giving water to all who are athirst. The yogi stands on the riverbank and scoops a handful of sacred water into her cupped hands, and in a worshipful gesture offers the water to the Sun, saying, "This knowledge has come through you; let me give it back to you." The knowledge of yoga ripples out into the world and returns to the earth as rain to be renewed again.

Yoga moves in circles. Your breath is a circle, wavelike, moving in toward you and away from you, in a circular motion. Your blood moves in circles around the body, from heart to peripheries and back to the heart again. The circle of yoga is one of giving and receiving.

In Yoga Sutra 1:12 Patanjali states, "The mind can reach the state of yoga through practice and detachment."[54] It can be alienating if we perceive detachment (*vairagya*) as cold, unfeeling, and disengaged. It's important to understand that being detached is not the same as being disinterested. The backbone of our yoga practice is always kindness and compassion, and it is this warmth that underpins the spirit of detached observation that we adopt during our practice of yoga.

Detachment allows us to stand back and observe the effects that our yoga practice is having upon us. We can then experiment and find out what works well and what doesn't. Paradoxically, by stepping back and observing what is happening, detachment enables us to connect with our body, mind, and emotions in a very intimate way.

There is a scientific side to yoga that is sometimes overlooked. The original yogis were scientists; they conducted experiments on their bodies and minds and then observed the results. Scientific observation requires an open mind, detachment, and letting go of preconceptions. Science will win the day if love takes it by the hand. Science + creativity + love = hope for the world.

Yoga is idealism, a vision of a better world: change, cooperation, and sharing resources. Kindness, giving it all away, circulating ideas: tweeting, blogging, texting communicating, rippling ideas across time and space. It is a force for change, a dancing revolution.

Change is in the air. Yoga is rebellious, radical. It makes waves—waves, rippling outward, creating the world anew. The tide comes in and the tide goes out. High tide, low tide. Sun on water. Moon on water. Yoga is generous and non-judgmental. With a wave-like rhythm, the breath moves in toward you and ripples out away from you.

In ancient times, in Hindu mythology, Gonika was a wise woman looking for someone to bequeath her knowledge of yoga upon. One day as she stood by a waterfall that flowed into a river, she scooped up a handful of river water into the cupped palms of her hands, and in a worshipful gesture offered the water to the Sun, saying, "This knowledge has come through you; let me give it back to you." Into her praying hands a serpent fell from heaven, and she called him Patanjali. *Pata* means both "serpent" and "fallen"; *anjali* means the worshipful gesture of her cupped hands.[55] The golden germ of yoga is said to have been born from the womb of the world. Yoga moves in circles.

---

54. T. K. V. Desikachar, *The Heart of Yoga: Developing Personal Practice* (Rochester, VT: Inner Traditions International, 1995), 153.

55. B. K. S. Iyengar, *The Tree of Yoga* (London: Thorsons, 2000), 74.

Yoga Inspired by Aquarius

Aquarius is a fixed, positive air sign. Traditionally, Aquarius was ruled by the planet Saturn; however, after the discovery of Uranus, it was assigned to that planet. Aquarian parts of the body are the shin, ankles, and circulatory system. Its color is electric blue. Key words are *detachedly* and *scientifically*.

Louis MacNeice, in his book *Astrology*, refers to Aquarius as the awakener and "the sign of the yogi through the development of spiritual consciousness through contemplation."[56] The association of the sign with the third eye, or *ajna,* chakra means it awakens the power of intuition. However, in Aquarius this intuitive insight is always backed up with rational, scientific knowledge. This Aquarian combination of a love for humanity, intuition, and evidence-based scientific knowledge could stand us in good stead as we grapple with modern dilemmas such as climate change and global warming.

The rulership of Uranus means that Aquarius is a rebel and likes to make waves. Aquarius is an idealistic sign that wants to change the world. The slogan "If I can't dance, it's not my revolution" was emblazoned across feminist T-shirts in the 1970s, and it is attributed to the anarchist, political activist, and writer Emma Goldman.[57] In Eastern religions the heartbeat is referred to as a mystic dance of life going on inside the body. In India the dancing Shiva was said to dwell at the beating heart of the cosmos.[58]

Aquarius-Inspired Yoga Practice

The heart is at the center of the circulatory system, which is assigned to Aquarius, and this provided me with the motif for the Aquarius-inspired yoga practice that follows. Consequently, the practice has a circular feel, echoing the other Aquarius theme of waves that ripples through the practice.

In Sanskrit Aquarius was *Khumba*, the pot, and although Aquarius is an air sign, its symbol is the water bearer. There is a real generosity within the imagery of the water bearer, bestowing the blessing of water upon all of humanity, regardless of their perceived merit. Its glyph, which is two wavy lines representing waves, adds to the watery feel of the sign. I have incorporated this in the Aquarius-inspired yoga practice that follows with the use of wavelike movements that ripple through the body. We use yoga

---

56. MacNeice, *Astrology*, 103.

57. Alix Kates Shulman, "Dances with Feminists," The Emma Goldman Papers, University of California, Berkeley Library, originally published in *Women's Review of Books* 9, no. 3 (December 1991), http://www.lib.berkeley.edu/goldman/Features/danceswithfeminists.html.

58. Walker, *The Woman's Encyclopedia of Myths and Secrets*, 376.

movements that flow into each other in a wavelike fashion, and there is an emphasis on observing the wavelike motion of the breath. Your breath is a wave, rising and falling, ebbing and flowing. The Sun, the Moon, the stars, and the Earth are all there in every breath you take. Wave upon wave, circles within circles, like a cosmic mandala.

The affirmation we use in the practice is *The wave of the breath ripples through me.* It can be coordinated with the breath:

Inhale: The wave of the breath

Exhale: Ripples through me

Allow 20 to 30 minutes.

1. Wavelike breathing

Find yourself a comfortable lying position. Bring your awareness to the natural rhythm of the flow of your breath. Over several breaths silently repeat this phrase: *The wave of the breath ripples through me.*

Now imagine that you are on the seashore, watching the waves rising and falling. Keep the image of the sea in your mind, and at the same time bring your awareness back to the natural flow of the breath. Notice the wavelike quality of the ebb and flow of your breath. Every so often return to the phrase *The wave of the breath ripples through me.*

Throughout the following yoga practice, keep bringing your awareness back to the wavelike quality of your breathing.

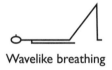

Wavelike breathing

2. Pelvic rocking

Lie on your back, both knees bent and both feet on the floor, about hip width apart. Gently rock your pelvis back and forth. Exhale and tuck the tailbone under. The back of the waist imprints into the floor and the lower abs contract. Inhale, your tailbone rocking toward the floor, the back of the waist arching up away from the floor, and the tummy sticking out. Continue gently rocking between these two movements. Cultivate a wavelike quality to the movement and coordinate it with the breath.

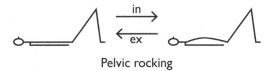

Pelvic rocking

3. Pelvic rocking and arm movements

Continue gently rocking your pelvis back and forth, and as you inhale, raise both arms above your head onto the floor behind you. As you exhale, lower the arms back to the sides. You can silently coordinate the breath and movement with the affirmation. Inhale and affirm, *The wave of the breath*. Exhale and affirm, *Ripples through me*. Repeat 6 times.

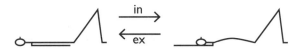

Pelvic rocking and arm movements

4. Cat Pose (Marjaryasana) *into* Cow Pose (Bitilasana)

Come onto all fours and begin by gently rocking the pelvis back and forth. Cultivate a wavelike quality to the movement and coordinate it with the breathing. Gradually shift from pelvic rocking into Cat Pose (*Marjaryasana*) and then into Cow Pose (*Bitilasana*). Exhale and round the back up like an angry cat. Inhale into Cow Pose, arching the back, lifting the chest up and away from the belly, and looking up slightly. Alternate between these two positions, rounding and arching the back. Repeat 8 times. (If you have a back problem, don't arch the back.)

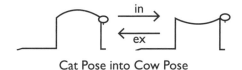

Cat Pose into Cow Pose

5. Cat Pose with leg movements (Marjaryasana *variation*)

Start on all fours. Exhale, rounding the back up and bringing one knee toward the head. Inhale, straightening the leg out behind you and keeping the pelvis level. Repeat 6 times on this side. Cultivate a wavelike feel to the movement and coordinate it with the breathing. Repeat on the other side.

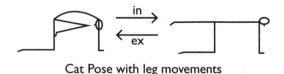

Cat Pose with leg movements

6. *Wavelike Lunge Pose* (Anjaneyasana *variation*)

From Cat Pose move your right foot forward until it is between your hands. Inhaling, come up onto your fingertips, extending through the length of the spine. Exhaling, lower your torso down toward your right thigh. With a wavelike motion alternate between these two movements 6 times. Then repeat on the other side.

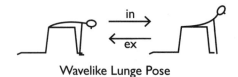

Wavelike Lunge Pose

7. *Lunge Pose with arm movements* (Anjaneyasana *variation*)

Come to tall kneeling. Take your right foot forward and bend the knee, bringing the knee over the ankle. Rest your fingertips lightly on your ears, elbows out to the side. Exhale, bringing the elbows to point to the front and down, rounding the upper back, and looking down. Inhaling, open the elbows, lift the chest, and look up slightly. Repeat 4 times and then stay in the open-chest position for a few breaths. Repeat on the other side.

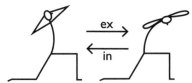

Lunge Pose with arm movements

8. *Downward-Facing Dog Pose* (Adho Mukha Svanasana) *into Standing Forward Bend* (Uttanasana)

From the Lunge Pose (*Anjaneyasana*), come back onto all-fours, turn the toes under and move into Downward-Facing Dog Pose (*Adho Mukha Svanasana*). Stay here for a few breaths. Then walk the hands back to the feet, coming into a Standing Forward Bend (*Uttanasana*). Stay here for a few breaths. To ease the pose, bend the knees more. Slowly uncurl, coming back up to standing.

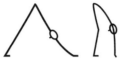

Downward-Facing Dog Pose into Standing Forward Bend

9. Mountain Pose (Tadasana) *with wavelike breathing*

Stand tall, feet parallel and about hip width apart. Notice the wavelike quality of the ebb and flow of your breath. Over several breaths silently repeat the phrase *The wave of the breath ripples through me.*

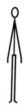

Mountain Pose with wavelike breathing

10. Warrior Pose (Virabhadrasana) *variation into Intense Side Stretch Pose* (Parsvottanasana) *variation*

Stand tall, feet hip width apart and both hands resting on the belly. Step one foot forward. Inhale, taking the arms out to the side and bending the front knee. Exhale, bending forward over the bent front leg and sweeping both arms behind the back. Inhale, coming back up and sweeping arms out to the side. Exhale, straightening the front leg and returning the hands to the belly. Repeat 4 times with a wavelike motion, and then repeat on the other side. On the final time in Intense Side Stretch Pose (*Parsvottanasana*), place both hands on the floor, on either side of the front foot, and step back into Downward-Facing Dog Pose (*Adho Mukha Svanasana*).

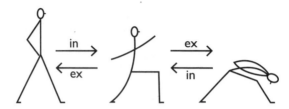

Warrior Pose variation into Intense Side Stretch Pose variation

11. *Downward-Facing Dog Pose* (Adho Mukha Svanasana) *into Plank Pose* (Chaturanga Dandasana)

Stay for a few breaths in Downward-Facing Dog Pose (*Adho Mukha Svanasana*). Then lower yourself down into Plank Pose (*Chaturanga Dandasana*) and stay for a few breaths.

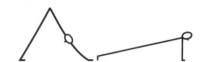

Downward-Facing Dog Pose into Plank Pose

12. *Child's Pose* (Balasana)

From Plank Pose (*Chaturanga Dandasana*) drop the knees to the floor, sitting back into Child's Pose (*Balasana*). Rest here for a few breaths.

Child's Pose

13. *Child's Pose* (Balasana) *into Upward-Facing Dog Pose* (Urdhva Mukha Svanasana)

From Child's Pose (*Balasana*) stretch the arms out along the floor. Inhale, moving forward into Upward-Facing Dog Pose (*Urdhva Mukha Svanasana*), arching your back, and keeping your knees on the floor. Exhale back into Child's Pose. You can silently coordinate the breath with the affirmation. Inhale and affirm, *The wave of the breath.* Exhale and affirm, *Ripples through me.* Repeat 6 times as you move between the two poses.

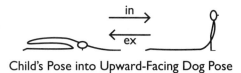

Child's Pose into Upward-Facing Dog Pose

14. *Boat Pose* (Navasana)

Come to sitting, legs outstretched in front of you, knees bent, and heels resting on the floor. Lean backward slightly, keeping a long back, with your head and neck in line with the spine and your lower abs gently pulling back toward the spine. Lift the heels from the floor and raise the legs to make a V shape out of your body. For an easier pose keep the legs slightly bent, or for more of a challenge straighten the legs. Do not round the back. As you hold the pose silently repeat this affirmation: *The wave of the breath ripples through me.*

Boat Pose

15. *Bridge Pose* (Setu Bandhasana) *into Curl-Up*

Lie on your back; knees bent, feet on the floor, hip width apart; arms by your sides. Inhale: peel your back from the floor, taking your arms overhead onto the floor behind you, coming into Bridge Pose (*Setu Bandhasana*). Exhale: lower the back, returning the arms back to the sides. Still exhaling (or take an extra breath), curl up into a ball, bringing the knees to the chest and the hands to the knees, and curling the head and shoulders off the floor into a curl-up. Inhale and come back to the starting position. Stay for one breath and then repeat the entire sequence. Aim to cultivate a wavelike quality to your movements, coordinating them with the breath. Repeat 4 to 6 times..

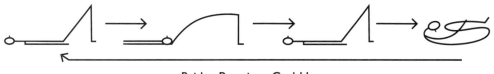

Bridge Pose into Curl-Up

16. Supine Twist (Jathara Parivrtti)

Lie on your back, knees bent, feet together, arms out to the sides at shoulder height, and palms facing down. Bring both knees onto your chest (for an easier pose keep both feet on the floor). Exhaling, lower both knees down toward the floor on the left and turn the head gently to the right. Inhale and return to center. With each exhale silently repeat the mantra *Vam* (pronounced *vum*). Allow your movements to be flowing and watery. Repeat 6 times on each side, alternating sides.

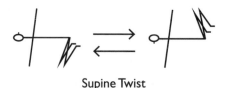

Supine Twist

17. Knees-to-Chest Pose (Apanasana)

Hug the knees into the chest. Rest here for a few breaths.

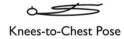

Knees-to-Chest Pose

18. Knees-to-Chest Pose (Apanasana) into leg stretch

Bring both knees onto your chest. Inhale and straighten your legs vertically, heels toward the ceiling. Take your arms out to the side, just below shoulder height, with the palms facing up. Exhaling, bring the knees back to the chest and the hands back to the knees. You can silently coordinate the breath with the affirmation. Inhale and affirm, *The wave of the breath.* Exhale and affirm, *Ripples through me.* Repeat 4 to 6 times. *Finish here or move on to step 19.*

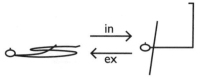

Knees-to-Chest Pose into leg stretch

19. Wavelike Breathing Exercise

If you have time, do the Wavelike Breathing Exercise that follows or the shortened version in step 1.

Aquarius-Inspired Yoga Practice Overview

1. Wavelike breathing. *The wave of the breath ripples through me.*

2. Pelvic rocking.

3. Pelvic rocking and arm movements. Inhale: *The wave of the breath.* Exhale: *Ripples through me.* Repeat × 6.

4. Cat Pose into Cow Pose × 8.

5. Cat Pose with leg movements × 6. Repeat on other side.

6. Wavelike Lunge Pose × 6. Repeat on other side.

7. Lunge Pose with arm movements × 4. Repeat on other side.

8. Downward-Facing Dog Pose into Standing Forward Bend. Stay for a few breaths in each pose.

9. Mountain Pose with wavelike breathing. *The wave of the breath ripples through me.*

10. Warrior Pose variation into Intense Side Stretch Pose variation × 4. Repeat on other side.

11. Downward-Facing Dog Pose into Plank Pose. Stay for a few breaths in each pose.

12. Child's Pose. Rest for a few breaths.

13. Child's Pose into Upward-Facing Dog Pose. Inhale: *The wave of the breath.* Exhale: *Ripples through me.* Repeat 6 times.

14. Boat Pose. Stay a few breaths. Repeat affirmation: *The wave of the breath ripples through me.*

15. Bridge Pose into Curl-Up × 4–6.

16. Supine Twist × 6 each side. On exhale mantra: *Vam.*

17. Knees-to-Chest Pose. Rest a few breaths.

18. Knees-to-Chest Pose into leg stretch. Inhale: *The wave of the breath.* Exhale: *Ripples through me.* Repeat × 4–6. *Finish here or move on to step 19 if time.*

19. Wavelike Breathing Exercise.

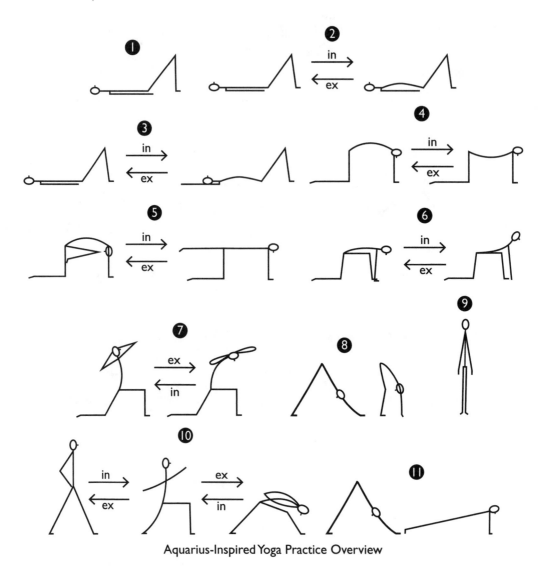

Aquarius-Inspired Yoga Practice Overview

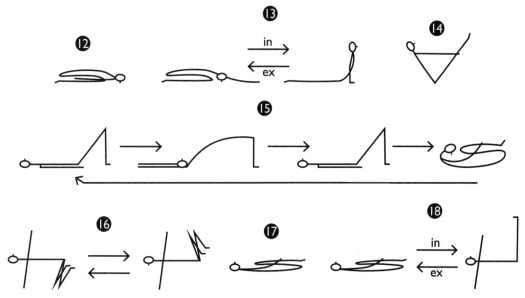

Aquarius-Inspired Yoga Practice Overview (continued)

EXERCISE

Wavelike Breathing

Aquarius is the sign of the rebel. Today's idealistic activists often suffer from burnout as they make waves and try to change the world for the better. The Wavelike Breathing Exercise is the perfect antidote to this exhaustion and gets you dancing with life again. It also fits in with the Aquarian themes of water and waves.

This exercise helps you restore a natural, healthy rhythm to your breathing. It has a calming, balancing, gently energizing effect. It helps you feel a connection with nature and tap into the incredible healing power of the breath. It is a very effective way of restoring your equilibrium if you've been through a time of upheaval or are feeling unsettled. It helps you accept change more willingly and to go with the ebb and flow of life.

Allow 10 to 15 minutes for this exercise.

Find yourself a comfortable position, either sitting or lying. Be aware of the support of the earth beneath you. Observe the downward pull of gravity and its effect upon your body. Picture the Moon in the sky above; remember that the Moon exerts gravitational pull upon the oceans of the Earth. Picture the Sun in the sky. Hold in your mind's eye an awareness of the Sun, the Moon, and the Earth, all in their own way influencing your body and the world around you.

Now bring your awareness to the natural rhythm of the flow of your breath. Simply observe the breath without controlling or shaping it. Particularly be aware of your thoracic breathing. Be aware of the chest and the movement of the rib-cage with every in- and out-breath. See if you can pinpoint where the fulcrum of thoracic breathing is located. The fulcrum is the still point, rather like the hinge on a door. Be aware of the thoracic breathing and be aware of a crystalline stillness all round you. You are aware of movement and you are aware of stillness.

Over several breaths silently repeat this phrase: *The wave of the breath ripples through me.* If you wish you can coordinate the phrase with the breathing:

Inhale: The wave of the breath

Exhale: Ripples through me

Now imagine that you are on the seashore observing the rising and falling of the waves. Imagine you can hear the sound of sea. In your mind's eye watch the ebb and flow of the waves as they lap against the shore. Keep the image of the sea in your mind, and at the same time bring your awareness back to the natural flow of the breath. Be aware of the sound of the breath, which is like the sound of the sea in a shell when it is held to the ear. Notice the wavelike quality of the ebb and flow of your breath. Every so often return to the phrase:

Inhale: The wave of the breath

Exhale: Ripples through me

Let go of visualizing the sea and come back to simply observing the natural ebb and flow of the breath. Imagine that around you there is a huge ocean of air and that with each breath the air moves through you in a wavelike motion, creating a ripple throughout the body. Observe the ripple effect of the air moving through your body with each breath in and out. Allow yourself to be moved by the breath. Feel the movement and at the same time be aware of a crystalline stillness, which is like the canvas through which the air moves.

When you feel ready, let go of observing the wavelike quality of the breath. Feel the support of the earth beneath you; feel the space around you; become aware of your surroundings; notice the sounds inside the room and outside the room. Observe the effect that the wavelike breathing has had upon you. Remind yourself that at any point in the day or night you can tune in to the wavelike quality of the breath and the crystalline stillness around you.

Aquarius-Inspired Meditation Questions

See chapter 1 for guidance on how to use the meditation questions. The theme for Aquarius is "idealism, detachment, science, and love."

- If I had been granted three wishes to make the world a better place, what would I wish for?
  - What small steps could I take to make this ideal world become a reality?
- What are my feelings about the yoga concept of detachment?
  - How does standing back and observing the effect my yoga practice is having on me benefit my practice?
  - Am I able to apply the same skills of detached observation to my daily life and so see the bigger picture?
  - How do I ensure that my detached attitude is infused with warmth and kindness and doesn't come across as being disinterested?
- How might a good knowledge of science and technology help me in my yoga practice and in my life?
  - Are there any new scientific or technical skills that I would like to learn?
- How would finding out more about the mechanics of breathing and the circulatory system benefit my yoga practice?
- How do I feel about getting older?
  - What can I learn from the wisdom of older people in my life?
  - Do I know an older person who would benefit from a "good listening to"?
- How would an understanding of the cycles of the natural world help me understand my own natural rhythms and cycles better?
- What ideas do I have for committing random acts of kindness?

CHAPTER 15

Diving Deep to Find Self-Knowledge

Pisces

February 19–March 20

Attune yourself to the circular flow of life, and come face to face with love.

Yoga works the miracle of relaxing the body. Like a dance of the seven veils, layer upon layer of tension is uncovered and released. This unlocking of tension helps us peep behind the veil of the subconscious mind. An example of this is when you do an early morning yoga practice and forgotten fragments of a dream float up like air bubbles from your subconscious into your conscious mind. *Revelation* comes from Latin and means "to draw back the veil."

Hidden within each of us are worlds within worlds. Sometimes we abandon our self to the periphery of our life and become a planet orbiting someone else's sun. Hidden forces can exert a gravitational pull on us, pulling the path of our life out of orbit. We all carry in our heart influences from the past: for example, a kind grandparent, a critical parent, or an overly strict teacher. Hidden and out of view, they carry on exerting

225

veiled strength from behind the scenes, sometimes benevolent and sometimes destructive. Yoga helps us peep behind the veil and bring these influences out into the light so we can work with them.

At times we turn to yoga feeling like we are stuck in a maze. We have no idea how to get out. It's easy to panic when we feel trapped, which makes us feel even more puzzled about how to escape. Yoga calms the mind and lifts the fog, and a way forward is revealed. The veil is lifted, and our inner, intuitive vison sees the bigger picture.

Yoga is a rainbow bridge uniting heaven and earth. It celebrates an embodied spirituality lived out in cycles. The Sun rises, the Sun sets, and the next morning rises again. We are born, we live our life, we die, and perhaps like the Sun we are reborn. Winter gives way to spring.

Look at the night sky: each pinprick of light could be a remote galaxy containing millions of stars. Keep a spacious and open mind. You don't need to rise above the everyday world simply work with it. Life is the guru. Surrender to life as it is. The silver thread that unites the waxing and waning Moon is the thread of love. Each ending is a new beginning.

When you can stay present to your life—not pushing it away, but surrounding it with love, compassion, and acceptance—this is the beginning of an authentic spiritual practice. When you can welcome light and dark, pleasant and unpleasant, waxing and waning, you come face to face with love.

At first staying present to your life as it is in the here and now is a discipline, but eventually love takes over. What starts off as hard graft and unrelenting practice turns into a love that is a real living presence. You can't make it happen; it's a gift. When it comes, it's strong enough to carry all your pain, as if you are wrapped in a cloak of warmth, safety, and love.

Live skillfully and with kindness. Be prepared to work with the limitations that are part of life and at the same time seek out and enjoy the beauty of life.

Outside dappled sunlight and shadow dance on the path. At the center of the mandala is the tree of life. Its roots go deep down into the earth and its branches reach up to the heavens. On one side of the tree is a moonlit, starry night and on the other brilliant sunshine.

Yoga Inspired by Pisces

Pisces is a mutable, negative water sign ruled by the planet Neptune. Its symbol is two fishes swimming in opposite directions. The feet and lymphatic system are the parts of the body assigned to it. Its metal is tin, and its color is sea green.

Some consider that with Pisces we have reached the highest point of yoga or spiritual consciousness.[59] It's a sign that is associated with the intangible, the spiritual, and the psychic. It is the most fluid of all the signs, with the water of Pisces being the water of the sea, infinitely deep and boundless.

The rulership of Neptune gives a depth and mystery to the sign. Key words of this planet are *nebulousness* and *impressionability*. It has to do with what hides itself from view and veiled strength from behind the scenes; this is because it was only discovered because its pull altered the regular path of Uranus. It can be revealing to explore in our own lives what are the hidden influences exerting a gravitational pull upon us and perhaps distorting our trajectory. Are there hidden players pulling our strings? Yoga helps us gain access to our subconscious; for example, in meditation we dive deep into the ocean of our mind and this can shed light on what was previously hidden from view. Once we are aware of these nebulous influences, we can either accept them, if they are benevolent, or change them if they are pulling us in a direction we don't want to go.

The feet are the part of the body assigned to Pisces. All over India the footprints of the Buddha are worshipped at holy shrines. In ancient times there were stones dedicated to Isis and Venus marked with footprints, meaning "I have been here." Egyptians, Babylonians, and other ancient peoples considered it essential to step on sacred ground with bare feet in order to absorb the holy influences.[60] Dedicating a yoga practice to focusing on the feet is always fruitful and can incorporate elements such as grounding, alignment, rootedness, connection to the earth, the pull of gravity, and finding support from the earth beneath our feet.

The Pisces glyph represents two crescent moons: one waxing and one waning. Originally, the glyph meant the waxing and waning of each life in cycles defined by the Moon.[61] The Sanskrit name for the constellation of Pisces was *Mina*, which means fish, and the glyph is sometimes interpreted as two fishes pulling in opposite directions, one representing the physical side of our nature and one representing the spiritual side. In

---

59. MacNeice, *Astrology*, 105.

60. Walker, *The Woman's Dictionary of Symbols and Sacred Objects*, 309.

61. Walker, *The Woman's Dictionary of Symbols and Sacred Objects*, 293.

yoga terms this would be the tension between *prakriti* (matter) and *purusha* (spirit). I prefer to see the thread that joins the two fishes as an umbilical cord that nourishes both spirit and matter, rather than the two working against each other.

Pisces-Inspired Yoga Practice

The Pisces glyph was my inspiration for the Pisces-inspired yoga practice that follows. The glyph encapsulates that just-before moment: the moment just before a flower opens, just before the New Moon is visible in the sky, just before sunrise, just before a baby opens its eyes and sees daylight for the first time.

The glyph's waxing and waning Moon represents the cyclical nature of life, where every ending is a new beginning. In the yoga practice, this led me to focus on the cycle of the breath, noticing where each part of the breath begins and ends, as well as observing the spaces between one breath ending and the next breath beginning. This focus gives a deeply meditative quality to the practice.

The practice is relaxing and energizing, grounding and elevating. It promotes stability, resilience, and an ability to flow with the ebb and flow of life. It provides an opportunity for a deep and profound healing to occur on both a physical and emotional level. It helps promote a healthy breathing pattern.

The affirmation we use in the practice is *A flower blossoms with each breath.* It can be coordinated with the breath:

Inhale: A flower blossoms

Exhale: With each breath

Allow 20 to 30 minutes.

1. Circular breathing and Pisces glyph visualization

Begin your practice lying down in a comfortable position. In your mind's eye visualize the Pisces glyph. Hold this image in your mind as you begin to follow the natural flow of your breath. As you observe the breath, notice where your inhalation begins and where it ends. Notice where your exhalation begins and where it ends. Be aware of the spaces between the breath. Notice the space between the end of the inhalation and the beginning of the exhalation, and the space between the end of the exhalation and the beginning of the next inhalation. Observe the circular nature of the breath, in which each ending is a new beginning. During this yoga practice, keep coming back to this focus on circular breathing and picturing the Pisces glyph.

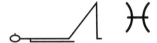

Circular breathing and Pisces glyph visualization

2. Blossoming feet visualization

During this practice, we focus on the feet, as they are the part of the body assigned to Pisces. Lying on your back, bend your knees, both feet on the floor and about hip width apart. Bring your awareness to the soles of your feet and picture a flower at the center of the foot. Imagine that each of your exhalations travels all the way down to the feet, and at the end of the exhalation there is a sense of opening and blossoming at the soles of the feet. During the practice, come back to an awareness of the feet blossoming on the exhalation as you hold each yoga pose. Then, silently repeat the affirmation a few times: *A flower blossoms with each breath.*

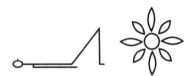

Blossoming feet visualization

3. Knees-to-Chest Pose (Apanasana) *into leg stretch*

Bring both knees onto your chest. Inhale and straighten your legs vertically, heels toward the ceiling, and take your arms out to the side just below shoulder height, palms facing up. Exhaling, bring knees back to chest and hands back to knees. You can silently coordinate the breath and movement with the affirmation. Inhale and affirm, *A flower blossoms.* Exhale and affirm, *With each breath.* Repeat 4 to 6 times.

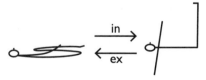

Knees-to-Chest Pose into leg stretch

4. Supine Tree Pose (Vrksasana supine)

Lie on your back, legs outstretched along the floor. Bring the sole of your left foot to rest on the inner right thigh; allow the left knee to rotate out to the side (to ease the pose put a support under the knee). Take the arms up above the head and bring the fingertips lightly together (to ease the pose have the arms shoulder width apart or wider). Stay here for a few breaths. Repeat on the other side.

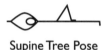

Supine Tree Pose

5. Cat Pose (Marjaryasana) into Cow Pose (Bitilasana)

Come onto all fours. Bring your awareness to your feet. Picture a flower at the center of each foot. Imagine that each exhalation travels all the way down to the feet, and at the end of the exhalation there is a blossoming at the soles of the feet, an opening, like a big yawn. Then after a few breaths, begin to do Cat to Cow movements. Exhaling, round the back up like an angry cat. Inhale into Cow Pose (*Bitilasana*), arching the back, lifting the chest up and away from the belly, and looking up slightly. Alternate between these two positions, rounding and arching the back. Repeat 8 times. (If you have a back problem, don't arch the back.)

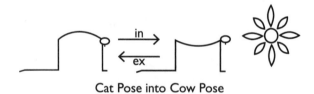

Cat Pose into Cow Pose

6. Downward-Facing Dog Pose (Adho Mukha Svanasana)

From the all fours position come into Downward-Facing Dog Pose (*Adho Mukha Svanasana*). Bring your awareness to your feet. Picture a flower at the center of each foot. Imagine that each exhalation travels all the way down to the feet, and at the end of the exhalation there is a blossoming in the soles of the feet. Stay here for a few breaths and then lower down back to all fours, ready for the next pose.

Downward-Facing Dog Pose

7. Cat Pose (Marjaryasana) *into* Child's Pose (Balasana)

From all fours, exhale and lower the bottom to the heels and the head to the floor into Child's Pose (*Balasana*). Inhale and come back up to all fours. Silently coordinate the breath and movement with the affirmation. Inhale and affirm, *A flower blossoms.* Exhale and affirm, *With each breath.* Repeat 6 times.

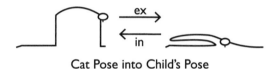

Cat Pose into Child's Pose

8. The Moonlit Tree Sequence

Follow these steps to perform the Moonlit Tree Sequence:

8a. Child's Pose (Balasana)

Stay here for a few breaths with the arms relaxed by the sides.

Child's Pose

8b. Sitting kneeling to Standing Forward Bend (Uttanasana)

Come to sitting kneeling, place the palms of the hands on the floor just in front of the knees, turn the toes under, and push yourself back into a relaxed Standing Forward Bend position (*Uttanasana*).

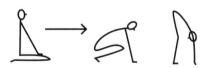

Sitting kneeling to Standing Forward Bend

8c. Standing Forward Bend (Uttanasana), bend knees and arch back

Stay in the Standing Forward Bend (*Uttanasana*) for a few breaths. Then, inhaling, bend the knees and arch the back. Exhaling, come back down into the forward bend. Repeat 4 times.

Standing Forward Bend, bend knees and arch back

8d. Standing with raised arms

Come back up to standing, raising the arms up above the head.

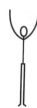

Standing with raised arms

8e. Dynamic Mini Squat

Stand tall, feet hip width apart and parallel, arms raised forward at just below shoulder height, palms facing down. Exhaling, bend the knees, coming into a mini-squat, and sweep the arms behind you. Inhaling, straighten the legs and bring the arms forward again. Repeat 4 times.

Dynamic Mini Squat

8f. Standing knee to chest

Hug your left knee into the chest.

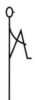

Standing knee to chest

8g. Tree Pose (Vrksasana) *into Swaying Tree Pose* (Vrksasana *variation*)

Come into Tree Pose (*Vrksasana*), left foot resting on right thigh. Picture a tree in the moonlight. Then, still in Tree Pose, do a gentle side bend to the left (Swaying Tree Pose). Come back to center.

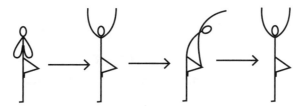

Tree Pose into Swaying Tree Pose

8h. Standing knee to chest

Hug your left knee to your chest. *Repeat 8f, 8g, and 8h on the other side.*

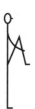

Standing knee to chest

8i. *Chair Pose* (Utkatasana)

Come into Chair Pose (*Utkatasana*). Stay for a few breaths.

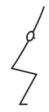

Chair Pose

8j. *Standing Forward Bend* (Uttanasana), *bend knees and arch back*

From Chair Pose (*Utkatasana*) melt down into a relaxed Standing Forward Bend (*Uttanasana*). Stay here for a few breaths. Inhaling, bend the knees and arch the back. Exhaling, come back down into the forward bend. Repeat 4 times.

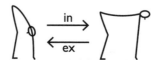

Standing Forward Bend, bend knees and arch back

8k. *Transition into Child's Pose* (Balasana)

Transition into Child's Pose (*Balasana*). From the Standing Forward Bend (*Uttanasana*), bend the knees, lower the bottom, and come back down into Child's Pose. Stay here for a few breaths and then repeat the sequence 2 to 3 more times.

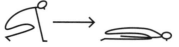

Transition into Child's Pose

9. *Blossoming feet visualization*

Lying on your back, bend your knees, both feet on the floor and about hip width apart. Bring your awareness to the soles of your feet. Picture a flower at the center of each foot. Imagine that each exhalation travels all the way down to the feet, and at the end of the exhalation there is a blossoming at the soles of the feet, an opening, like a big yawn. Then, silently repeat your affirmation a few times: *A flower blossoms with each breath.*

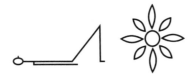

Blossoming feet visualization

10. *Bridge Pose with arm movements* (**Setu Bandhasana**)

Lie on your back, both knees bent, both feet on the floor hip width apart, and hands resting on your lower abdomen. Bring your awareness to your feet. Picture a flower at the center of each foot. Imagine that each exhalation travels all the way down to the feet, and at the end of the exhalation there is a blossoming in the soles of the feet. Inhaling, peel the back from the floor and come up into Bridge Pose, simultaneously taking the arms out to the sides and onto the floor, just below shoulder level, palms facing up. Exhaling, return to the starting position. You can silently coordinate the breath and movement with the affirmation. Inhale and affirm, *A flower blossoms.* Exhale and affirm, *With each breath.* Repeat 4 to 6 times.

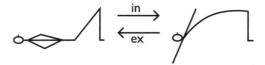

Bridge Pose with arm movements

11. *Knees-to-Chest Pose* (**Apanasana**) *into Full-Body Stretch*

Hug the knees into the chest. Rest here for a few breaths. Then have a full-body stretch, lengthening tall along the floor.

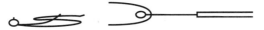

Knees-to-Chest Pose into Full-Body Stretch

12. *Circular breathing and Pisces glyph visualization*

Find a comfortable position lying down. In your mind's eye visualize the Pisces glyph. Hold this image in your mind as you begin to follow the natural flow of your breath. As you observe the breath, notice where your inhalation begins and where it ends. Notice where your exhalation begins and where it ends. Be aware of the spaces between the breath. Notice the space between the end of the inhalation and the beginning of the exhalation and the space between the end of the exhalation and the beginning of the next inhalation. Observe the circular nature of the breath, in which each ending is a new beginning.

You can either finish your practice here or go on to step 13.

Circular breathing and
Pisces glyph visualization

13. Simply Being Deep Relaxation

If you have time, do the Simply Being Deep Relaxation on page 238.

Pisces-Inspired Yoga Practice Overview

1. Circular breathing and Pisces glyph visualization.

2. Blossoming feet visualization.

3. Knees-to-Chest Pose into leg stretch × 4–6. Inhale: *A flower blossoms.* Exhale: *With each breath.*

4. Supine Tree Pose. Stay a few breaths.

5. Cat Pose into Cow Pose × 8 plus blossoming feet imagery.

6. Downward-Facing Dog Pose plus blossoming feet imagery.

7. Cat Pose into Child's Pose × 6. Inhale: *A flower blossoms.* Exhale: *With each breath.*

8. The Moonlit Tree Sequence:

   8a. Child's Pose. Stay for a few breaths.

   8b. Sitting kneeling to Standing Forward Bend.

   8c. Standing Forward Bend. Bend knees and arch back × 4.

   8d. Come back up to standing, raising the arms up above the head.

   8e. Dynamic Mini Squat × 4.

   8f. Standing knee to chest.

   8g. Tree Pose into Swaying Tree.

   8h. Standing knee to chest.

   Repeat 8f, 8g, and 8h on the other side.

   8i. Chair Pose. Stay for a few breaths.

8j. Standing Forward Bend. Bend knees and arch back × 4.

8k. Bend the knees and transition into Child's Pose. Stay a few breaths.

Repeat sequence × 2–3.

9. Blossoming Feet Visualization.

10. Bridge Pose with arm movements × 4–6. Inhale: *A flower blossoms.*
Exhale: *With each breath.*

11. Knees-to-Chest Pose into Full-Body Stretch.

12. Circular breathing and Pisces glyph visualization.
Finish here or move on to step 13.

13. Simply Being Deep Relaxation.

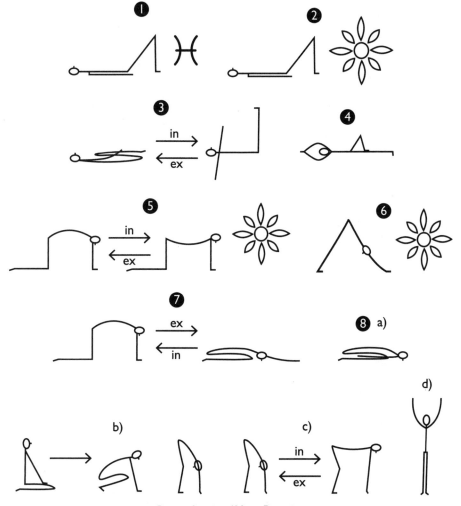

Pisces-Inspired Yoga Practice

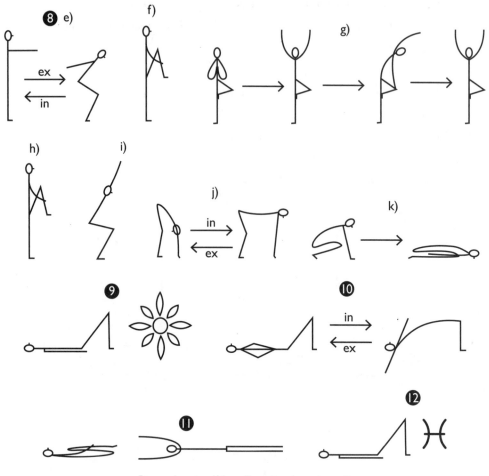

Pisces-Inspired Yoga Practice (continued)

RELAXATION

The Simply Being Deep Relaxation

The Pisces glyph teaches us to relax into the ebb and flow of life. In the same way, this relaxation teaches us to relax into the rising and falling of thoughts, feelings, and passing bodily sensations. Pisces is a watery sign, as deep as the sea, and as we let go into deeply relaxed states, we gain access to the depths of the mind. This also corresponds with the influence of Neptune, which is concerned with revealing what has been concealed and hidden and bringing it into the light of awareness.

The state of relaxation is a gift and not something that you can will into being by effort alone. In our everyday life off the yoga mat, problem-solving skills can be a great asset, but they're not the right tool for the job when it comes to relaxation. Relaxation flourishes when we let go of doing and slip into being mode.

Paradoxically, the more you *try* to relax, the more elusive relaxation becomes. When we set ourselves a goal of achieving a relaxed state, a discrepancy arises between where we are and where we want to get to. Consequently, a period of yoga relaxation in Relaxation Pose (*Savasana*) can become a battleground spent fighting off persistent thoughts, strong feelings, or physical discomfort. Counterintuitively, it's the effort of pushing away anything we perceive as an obstacle to relaxation that keeps us trapped in this perpetual cycle of tension. What we resist persists.

The Simply Being Deep Relaxation creates the right conditions for relaxation to be realized. It's a method that teaches you how to relax into the present moment and to accept yourself as you are. It trains you to cultivate qualities that will help you to relax, such as presence, acceptance, being non-judgmental, curiosity, and compassion. Once you let go of the effort and struggle to relax, you may well find that you get into the habit of dropping quickly and easily into a deeply relaxed state.

The method that we use in this relaxation is a meditation technique called "choiceless awareness." Instead of setting ourselves the goal of relaxing, we set the intention of simply being present to whatever arises. Choiceless awareness is like sitting on the banks of a river and watching passing debris floating by. The river is the flow of your consciousness and the objects floating by are thoughts, feelings, and physical sensations. Your aim is to simply observe the detritus carried along by the river, such as an autumn leaf, a branch fallen from a tree, a rusty can, an old boot, ducks, swans, and boats going by. All these things come and go, but the flow of the river is constant.

Set a timer for between 5 and 20 minutes and commit to stay present to whatever arises (choiceless awareness) for that specific amount of time.

Find yourself a comfortable position lying down in Relaxation Pose (*Sava-sana*). If you have a back problem, bend your knees and keep feet flat on the floor, or place a pillow under your knees and rest your legs straight, hip width apart.

Although we are not "trying" to relax, the body is more likely to relax if you place it in an optimum position to promote relaxation. Check that you're symmetrically arranged around the midline of the spine. Relax your shoulders down away from the ears. Unclench the jaw by slightly parting the teeth. Relax the face with a half smile. If your arms are by your sides, then have the palms facing upward and the fingers lightly curled, or rest your hands on your belly. Notice where your body is in contact with the floor and allow yourself to let go into the support of the earth.

Become aware of the natural flow of your breath. Don't try to impose a pattern on the breathing; simply observe it. If you rest your awareness on the movement of the breath at the belly, it will have a relaxing effect. You can always come back to this anchor of the breath at the belly at any point during this relaxation/meditation.

Now you are ready to practice choiceless awareness. Start by setting your intention to let go of trying to relax and aim to simply be present to your experience as it arises from moment to moment. The "object" of your meditation is whatever comes up most strongly for you, whether it's a thought, a feeling, an irritating noise, or a physical sensation. Whatever comes up most strongly becomes your focus, the thing that you pay attention to. Let's have a look at what might arise for you during this period of choiceless awareness and the best way to work with it by adopting an attitude of approach rather than avoidance.

Physical Tension: It's tempting to jump right in and to try to fix the problem by trying to make the tense area of the body relax. Instead try approaching physical sensations with curiosity. Notice how the sensations change from minute to minute, sometimes becoming more intense and at other times disappearing. Smile to the tense, uncomfortable part of your body; surround it with love and allow it to be exactly as it is in this moment. If the feelings get too intense, return to the anchor of observing your breath at the belly.

Persistent Thoughts: Although it's possible to cultivate a positive attitude, it isn't possible to control our thoughts. We can't decide to only think positive thoughts, and the effort to do so is very unrelaxing. Allow your thoughts to come and go. Observe them without getting too caught up in them. Notice the blue-sky space between thoughts. Smile to your thoughts, and surround them with love and kindness. If you need to take time out from observing thoughts, go back to the anchor of the breath.

Strong Emotions: Our emotions are like the weather; just as we can't decide whether it's going to be a sunny day, likewise we aren't able to choose our feelings. Allow the feelings to come and go, like clouds passing across a clear blue sky. Observe them with a compassionate, loving attitude, neither pushing them away nor getting too tangled up in them. If you need to take time out from being present to feelings, go back to the anchor of the breath.

Distracting Noise: That's lucky! You can meditate upon the sounds that arise and they become your object of meditation. Let go of judging sounds as pleasant or unpleasant. Just allow them to be as they are. Notice their timbre, volume, duration. Notice the silence between the sounds.

In choiceless awareness your "job" is simply to observe whatever comes up for you. So, if a persistent thought arises, don't push it away or get over-involved with it. Simply step back, observe it, and watch it rise, fall, and eventually pass away. The same applies to strong feelings, physical sensations, or even annoying sounds. Rather than seeing these as negative things that get in the way of your relaxation, allow them to become the thing that you observe, your teacher. Whatever comes up, step back, observe it, and surround it with love.

Approach whatever comes up with an accepting, non-judgmental attitude; observe it with curiosity, acceptance, and compassion. Allow it to be as it is. If painful feelings or thoughts arise, lovingly soothe them, cradling them and rocking them like a crying baby in arms. If at any point you feel overwhelmed by what's arising, come back to the anchor of observing the breath at the belly.

Once your timer has gone off, bring your awareness back to where your body is in contact with the floor or your support. Observe how you are feeling now and how the relaxation/meditation has affected you. Resolve to take any positive qualities you have developed, such as acceptance, patience, and compassion, back into your everyday life and the very next thing that you do today.

Pisces-Inspired Meditation Questions

See chapter 1 for guidance on how to use the meditation questions. The theme for this set of meditation questions is "uncovering hidden influences, navigating mazes, and going with the ebb and flow of life."

- What are the positive influences in my life that help me stay on course?
  - Who supports me and helps me keep on track?
- What are the negative influences that pull me off course?
  - Are any of these subtle and hidden, and if so, how could I bring them out into the light?
- When my life feels like a maze, what do I find are the best strategies for finding my way out?
  - What factors in my life do I find disorienting?
  - What factors help me navigate my way more effectively?
- In what ways am I aware of endings and new beginnings in my life?
  - In what ways am I aware of endings and new beginnings in the natural world around me?
- In my yoga practice what does observing the ebb and flow of the breath teach me?
  - In what ways are these lessons relevant to my everyday life?
- What is blossoming in my life right now?
  - What signs of new green shoots have I observed?
- At this time of equinox how does my yoga practice help me find balance in my life?

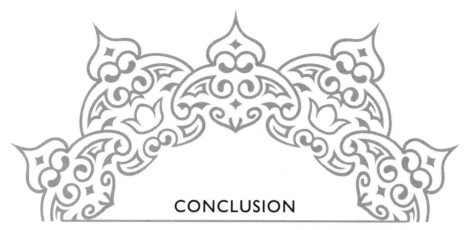

Our Pilgrimage around the Zodiac Wheel Continues

Thank you for joining me for one turn around the wheel of the zodiac. Although you have come to the end of this book, the journey continues. Every ending is a new beginning. Take some time now to pause and reflect on what you have learned from the book.

- What changes have occurred within you and your life over the course of reading this book?
- What are the skills and tools that you wish to take away from the book and use in your everyday life?
- How do you plan to move forward with your study of yoga and astrology?

Yoga is a circle, the year is a circle, and this book is circular too. Each time you return and reread a chapter in this book, the gift of yoga and the treasures of the zodiac will be there for you. Contained within each of the chapters of this book is the wisdom and healing power that is encapsulated in each of the zodiac signs. This combined with zodiac-inspired yoga practices has the potential to bring inspiration and transformation to your life. Over the years as you change and grow, so too will your appreciation and understanding of how best to use the zodiac and yoga treasures contained within these pages.

It is traditional at the end of a yoga practice to give thanks for the blessings that you have received and to dedicate the blessings to the benefit of all humanity. So, if it feels right, please send out a heartfelt wish that your friends, family, and wider community may all find their own way to healing, wisdom, self-knowledge, connection, love, and bliss, or whatever other blessings you wish to share with them.

The Tree of Life has her roots deep down in Mother Earth. Above, the black dome of the sky smiles down with stars. We also dedicate the blessings of our practice to the Earth. Astronauts looking down on planet Earth from space speak of feeling incredibly moved by the beauty and fragility of our planet as it spins in the darkness of space. The urgency of looking after the Earth with its finite resources dawns on them: there is no planet B. It's unlikely that you or I will travel to the Space Station, but as yogis we can train our mind's eye to take an astronaut's bird's-eye view of our beautiful planet. Our spiritual practice enables us to rise above the everyday and to see clearly what needs to be done to embody love in action. Look up to the stars for inspiration, but at same time recognize the treasure you have here on Earth.

The Sun is at the center, and around the Sun are the twelve signs of the zodiac. You are the Sun that has shone a light into each of the twelve signs revealing the treasure to be found within. Without you, without your sunlight, there is no life in the signs. It is you, your light, who have brought them to life and allowed them to shine. The purpose of our pilgrimage around the zodiac wheel has been to find the Sun at the center of our life, and now it's time for you to shine that light out into the world. Go shine!

Bibliography

Blake, William. "Auguries of Innocence." In *Poets of the English Language*. New York: Viking Press, 1950.

Brach, Tara. *Radical Acceptance: Embracing Your Life with the Heart of a Buddha*. New York: Bantam Dell, 2004.

Brandt Riske, Kris. *Complete Book of Astrology: The Easy Way to Learn Astrology*. Woodbury, MN: Llewellyn Publications, 2018.

Bruck, Mary T. *The Ladybird Book of the Night Sky*. Loughborough, England: Wills & Hepworth, 1965.

Campion, Nicholas. *A History of Western Astrology*. Vol. 1, *The Ancient World*. New York, NY: Bloomsbury Academic, 2015.

———. *A History of Western Astrology*. Vol. 2, *The Medieval and Modern Worlds*. New York: Bloomsbury Academic, 2013.

De Michelis, Elizabeth. *A History of Modern Yoga: Patanjali and Western Esotericism*. London: Continuum, 2005.

Denton, Lynn Teskey. *Female Ascetics in Hinduism*. Albany: State University of New York Press, 2004.

Desikachar, T. K. V. *The Heart of Yoga: Developing Personal Practice*. Rochester, VT: Inner Traditions International, 1995.

Eliade, Mircea. *Yoga: Immortality and Freedom*. Princeton, NJ: Princeton University Press, 1958.

Feuerstein, Georg. *Encyclopedic Dictionary of Yoga*. London: Unwin Hyman, 1990.

———. *The Yoga Tradition: Its History, Literature, Philosophy and Practice*. Prescott, AZ: Holm Press, 2001.

Goldberg, Natalie. *Writing Down the Bones: Freeing the Writer Within*. Boston, MA: Shambhala Publications, 1986.

Greene, Liz. *The Astrological World of Jung's* Liber Novus. London: Routledge, 2018.

———. *Jung's Studies in Astrology: Prophecy, Magic, and the Qualities of Time*. London: Routledge, 2018.

Gupta, Roxanne Kamayani. *A Yoga of Indian Classical Dance: The Yogini's Mirror*. Rochester, VT: Inner Traditions International, 2000.

Holm, Jean. *Women in Religion*. With John Bowler. New York: Continuum, 2004.

Hone, Margaret E. *The Modern Text-Book of Astrology*. London: L. N. Fowler & Co., 1975.

Iyengar, B. K. S. *The Tree of Yoga*. London: Thorsons, 2000.

Jung, C. G. *Jung on Astrology*. Edited by Safron Rossi and Keiron Le Grice. London: Routledge, 2018.

Kindred, Glennie. *The Alchemist's Journey: An Old System for a New Age*. London: Hay House UK, 2005.

Kornfield, Jack. *A Path with Heart*. London: Ebury Press, 2002.

Kraftsow, Gary. *Yoga for Transformation*. New York: Penguin, 2002.

MacNeice, Louis. *Astrology*. London: Bloomsbury, 1989.

Mayo, Jeff. *The Astrologer's Astronomical Handbook*. London: The Camelot Press, 1972.

Murdoch, Iris. *The Sea, the Sea*. London: Chatto and Windus, 1978. Reprint. London: Vintage, 1999. Citations refer to the Vintage edition.

Murray, William Hutchison. *The Scottish Himalayan Expedition*. London: J. M. Dent & Sons, 1951.

Nhat Hanh, Thich. *The Long Road Turns to Joy: A Guide to Walking Meditation*. Berkeley, CA: Parallax Press, 2011.

Pintchman, Tracy. *Women's Lives, Women's Rituals in the Hindu Tradition*. New York: Oxford University Press, 2007.

Roebuck, Valerie J. *The Circle of Stars: An Introduction to Indian Astrology*. Rockport, MA: Element, 1992.

Rumi. "The Guest House." In *The Essential Rumi*. Translated by Coleman Barks and John Moyne. San Francisco: Harper, 1997.

Sabatini, Sandra. *Breath: The Essence of Yoga; A Guide to Inner Stillness*. London, UK: Thorsons, 2000.

Shulman, Alix Kates. "Dances with Feminists." The Emma Goldman Papers. University of California, Berkeley Library. Originally published in Women's Review of Books 9, no. 3 (December 1991). http://www.lib.berkeley.edu/goldman/Features/danceswith feminists.html.

Simmer-Brown, Judith. *Dakini's Warm Breath: The Feminine Principle in Tibetan Buddhism*. Boston, MA: Shambhala Publications, 2003.

Stoler Miller, Barbara. *Yoga: Discipline of Freedom; The Yoga Sutra Attributed to Patanjali*. New York: Bantam Books, 1998.

Stone, Merlin. *When God Was a Woman*. Orlando, FL: Harcourt, 1976.

Walker, Barbara G. *The Woman's Dictionary of Symbols and Sacred Objects*. New York: HarperCollins, 1988.

———. *The Woman's Encyclopedia of Myths and Secrets*. New York: HarperCollins Publishers, 1983.

Recommended Resources

Astrology

See my bibliography for a list of the astrology books that I used when writing this book. Check out my website for ideas and inspiration for zodiac-inspired yoga practices: www.yogabythestars.com

Also, see the website of my publisher, Llewellyn Publications, as they have a comprehensive selection of books covering all aspects of astrology: www.llewellyn.com/browse_astrology.php

The *Earth Pathways Diary* includes UK sunrise, sunset, moonrise, and moonset times; moon phases and signs; and some astrological information: www.earthpathwaysdiary.uk

Stargazing

An internet search will find you a myriad of wonderful astronomy sites. Do some detective work and see what appeals to you. Be prepared to come across awe-inspiring pictures of our solar system and beyond! Below are some that I find useful:

www.darksky.org
www.stardate.org

Yoga Beginners

There are so many great yoga books out there, so go online and see what's available and what appeals to you. The ones below are user-friendly, and their approaches to yoga are similar to the one used in this book:

Lasater, Judith. *30 Essential Yoga Poses: For Beginning Students and Their Teachers.* Berkeley, CA: Rodmell Press, 2003.

Pierce, Margaret D., and Martin G. Pierce. *Yoga for Your Life: A Practice Manual of Breath and Movement for Every Body.* Portland, OR: Rudra Press, 1996.

Rountree, Sage. *Everyday Yoga: At-Home Routines to Enhance Fitness, Build Strength, and Restore Your Body.* Boulder, CO: Velopress, 2015.

There are lots of brilliant resources for beginners and more experienced students to be found online, so explore and see what's out there and what appeals to you. Also, ask your yoga friends for recommendations too. Below are some websites that I regularly use. Esther Ekhart's website is an invaluable resource for beginners and more experienced student:.

www. yogajournal.com

www.ekhartyoga.com

Yoga Practice

Below are some of my favorite yoga books. They are the ones I wouldn't lend out as I'm always referring to them:

Bennett, Bija. *Emotional Yoga: How the Body Can Heal the Mind.* London, UK: Bantam Books, 2002.

Farhi, Donna. *Yoga Mind, Body & Spirit: A Return to Wholeness.* New York: Henry Holt, 2000.

Kraftsow, Gary. *Yoga for Wellness: Healing with the Timeless Teachings of Viniyoga.* New York: Penguin, 1999.

Lee, Cyndi. *Yoga Body, Buddha Mind.* New York: Riverhead Books, 2004.

Powers, Sarah. *Insight Yoga.* Boston, MA: Shambhala Publications, 2008.

Sabatini, Sandra. *Breath: The Essence of Yoga; A Guide to Inner Stillness.* London, UK: Thorsons, 2000.

Scaravelli, Vanda. *Awakening the Spine: The Stress-Free New Yoga That Works with the Body to Restore Health, Vitality, and Energy.* New York: HarperCollins, 1991.

To Write to the Author

If you wish to contact the author or would like more information about this book, please write to the author in care of Llewellyn Worldwide Ltd. and we will forward your request. Both the author and publisher appreciate hearing from you and learning of your enjoyment of this book and how it has helped you. Llewellyn Worldwide Ltd. cannot guarantee that every letter written to the author can be answered, but all will be forwarded. Please write to:

Jilly Shipway
℅ Llewellyn Worldwide
2143 Wooddale Drive
Woodbury, MN 55125-2989

Please enclose a self-addressed stamped envelope for reply,
or $1.00 to cover costs. If outside the U.S.A., enclose
an international postal reply coupon.

Many of Llewellyn's authors have websites with additional information and resources. For more information, please visit our website at http://www.llewellyn.com.